Atlas of
HUMAN FEMALE
REPRODUCTIVE FUNCTION
Ovarian development to early embryogenesis
after *in vitro* fertilization

Dedicated to
Professor Pietro M Motta
1942–2002

Atlas of
HUMAN FEMALE REPRODUCTIVE FUNCTION

Ovarian development to early embryogenesis
after *in vitro* fertilization

Sayoko Makabe MD PhD
Department of Obstetrics and Gynecology
Toho University, Tokyo, Japan

and

Jonathan Van Blerkom PhD
Department of Molecular, Cellular and Developmental Biology
University of Colorado, Boulder, CO, USA
and Colorado Reproductive Endocrinology
Rose Medical Center, Denver, CO, USA

with the collaboration of

Stefania A Nottola MD PhD
Department of Human Anatomy
University of Rome 'La Sapienza', Rome, Italy

and

Tomonori Naguro PhD
Division of Genome Morphology
Tottori University, Yonago, Japan

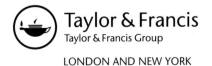

Taylor & Francis
Taylor & Francis Group

LONDON AND NEW YORK

© 2006 Taylor & Francis, an imprint of the Taylor & Francis Group

First published in the United Kingdom in 2006
by Taylor & Francis,
an imprint of the Taylor & Francis Group,
2 Park Square, Milton Park
Abingdon, Oxon OX14 4RN, UK

Tel.:   +44 (0) 20 7017 6000
Fax.:   +44 (0) 20 7017 6699
E-mail: info.medicine@tandf.co.uk
Website: http://www.tandf.co.uk/medicine

Although every effort has been made to ensure that all owners of copyright material have been acknowledged in this
publication, we would be glad to acknowledge in subsequent reprints or editions any omissions brought to our
attention.

British Library Cataloguing in Publication Data

Data available on application

Library of Congress Cataloging-in-Publication Data

Data available on application

ISBN 10: 1-84214-121-X
ISBN 13: 9-78-1-84214-121-2

Distributed in North and South America by

Taylor & Francis
2000 NW Corporate Blvd
Boca Raton, FL 33431, USA

Within Continental USA
Tel.: 800 272 7737; Fax.: 800 374 3401
Outside Continental USA
Tel.: 561 994 0555; Fax.: 561 361 6018
E-mail: orders@crcpress.com

Distributed in the rest of the world by
Thomson Publishing Services
Cheriton House
North Way
Andover, Hampshire SP10 5BE, UK
Tel.: +44 (0) 1264 332424
E-mail: salesorder.tandf@thomsonpublishingservices.co.uk

Composition by Parthenon Publishing
Printed and bound by T. G. Hostench S.A., Spain

Contents

Foreword

Divided into two sections, the first on the human ovary and the second on the mature oocyte and preimplantation embryo, this book brings together a welter of wonderful photographs on electron microscopy and a clear and detailed text taking the reader to the frontiers of knowledge on human follicles, oocytes and preimplantation embryos. It is dedicated to the late Pietro Motta, and reflects the astonishing standards of perfection in his books from Parthenon Publishing; sadly, there will be no more.

Section One on the human ovary initially salutes the pioneers de Graaf, van Horne, Malpighi and von Baer, then provides structural and ultrastructural aspects of ovarian dynamics and function in the adult. A well-written and masterly text and successive eye-catching illustrations offer a beautiful atlas of early development from primordial germ cells (PGCs) to the oogonia and oocytes, together with fresh outlooks on aspects of human *in vitro* fertilization (IVF). The authors stress how the origin, migration and settlement of PGCs have been well studied, yet major gaps still exist in our knowledge. How PGCs are formed remains a mystery, and how they separate from some by epiblast stages is unknown. Morphologically, they are found in the dorsal wall of the endodermal yolk sac as revealed in the sketches and illustrations of the developing human embryo. Light and electron microscopy, combined with excellent coloring, reveals them entering the yolk sac, moving passively to hindgut and dorsal mesentery and finally into the genital ridges. A large nucleus and few mitochondria characterize PGCs, and successive stages in their development by week 5 are detailed to reveal their association with somatic cells via gap junctions as visualized by sample fracture during transmission electron microscopy. Many of the beautiful illustra-tions take a full page, and each of them must have needed dedication and time to complete. A supportive text comments on ultrastructural and other aspects of the development of PGCs, their initial passive and later ameboid movements. Unsolved questions include how they know where to go and the underlying genetic control of these developmental stages and the components of extracellular matrix.

Equal authority and in brilliant color are applied throughout the text, including the settlement of PGCs in superficial ovarian layers of the human ovary at week 6. Their wanderings in and outside the ovary are described in relation to their structure, inclusive of their large nucleus, many mitochondria and great reductions in lipids and glycogen. Somatic components increase as PGCs multiply, and ovigerous sex cord-like structures form at week 7 to be followed by the delineation of cortex and medulla. Multiplying oogonia differentiate with few mito-chondria, an electron-dense granular substrate containing RNA and proteins, and also nuage which provides a cytoplasmic marker of developing germ-cell lineages. Between weeks 12 and 16, mesenchymal stromal cells and vessels have colonized both medulla and cortex, nests of germ cells have been formed and the sex cords are differentiating, as shown in immense detail. Notable intercellular bridges between oogonia and developing oocytes cells may facilitate exchanges between neighbors. Clear and informative illustrations display the early meiotic stages, their arrest at diplotene, and fine electron-dense threads in ooplasm which later shorten as chromosomes condense. Associations are shown between mitochondria and outer nuclear membranes, between chromosomes and the inner nuclear membrane, and as Balbiani's body is formed.

Flattened cells from ovigerous cords enclose nests of oogonia and oocytes to initiate oogenesis and folliculogenesis. The contentious origin of these cells and the nature of interstitial glandular cells, which may be steroid-producing cells, are discussed. Many of the numerous follicles (2 million in each ovary) seemingly undergo apoptosis, and others are seemingly exfoliated from (though still attached to) the ovarian surface in a process that continues until birth. Astonishingly, the hole-like structures shown in the surfaces of human ovaries at birth may be remnants of the passages where oocytes were expelled.

Phase 2 of the first section considers the adult human ovary and opens with mesothelial cells on its surface, their dynamic changes during the menstrual cycle, and their formation of surface papillae. Numerous resting and growing follicles are displayed, their primordial oocytes containing mitochondria, Golgi vesicles, endoplasmic reticulum, annulate amellae and Balbiani bodies. The zona pellucida is formed as cells surrounding the oocytes disperse while linked with the oocyte via microvilli passing through it to connect with Golgi complexes and mitochondria in ooplasm. A human follicle may require 100 days for its full development as its later stages, and perhaps early stages, require support from pituitary gonadotropins. Surrounding cells now become granulosa cells which proliferate, produce steroid hormones and growth factors and produce a fluid forming the follicular antrum. Illustrations reveal how preovulatory follicles expand, possess a distinct antrum, and how corona-cumulus cells surround the oocyte in an arc and form extensive cytoplasmic connections with it. Their granulosa cells in display reveal they are scattered and produce steroid hormones including progesterone, that many undergo apoptosis as ovulation approaches and their follicular membrane ruptures at ovulation to permit expulsion of the oocyte. Examples are shown of polycystic ovaries with numerous non-ovulated follicles and non-luteinizing unruptured follicles.

Section 2 phase 1 continues along similar themes and illustrations, stressing the modern significance of electron microscopy to clinical aspects of IVF which demands detailed knowledge of all preimplantation stages. The associated text does not shirk dealing with molecular biology and embryogenesis. Fundamental aspects of fertilization include the significance of the cortical granules, shown in clear detail by confocal microscopy, the numerous mitochondria and germinal vesicle breakdown induced by the mid-cycle LH surge or by administering hCG. Examples in text and images are provided to show how these systems can fail, or unexpected findings during IVF such as the fertilization of a germinal vesicle oocyte, and the formation of vacuoles in ooplasm. A semi-transparent disc-like structure surrounded by mitochondria is shown as an inherited cause of infertility. Examples of top-quality oocytes and their structure in successive illustrations include the structure of the meiotic spindle and its possible disorganization. The authors fully justify their assertion that transmission electron microscopy continues to identify and clarify subtle anomalies in human IVF embryos.

The same patterns of analysis continue to cover the preimplantation stages of development. New and dynamic aspects of development emerge such as the various phases of sperm entry, pronuclear formation and syngamy, which embrace highly significant aspects of inheritance. Numerous illustrations cover these and later stages to display sperm–zona interactions, post-fertilization spherical ridges in the zona pellucida and the attachment of too many spermatozoa to it. The detailed text continues to analyze the underlying factors producing superb pictures of these and other events, such as the acrosome reaction, time-lapse images, stunning images of the microtubular network, the spindle forming for the first cleavage division, and polarized nucleolar precursor bodies in fertilized oocytes. Brilliant colored images continue to impress accompanied by deep discussions on cleavage divisions and the blastocyst formation. Lovely examples reveal how mitochondria are inherited differentially by individual human 2-cell and 4-cell blastomeres, and how multiple or fragmented nuclei and cytoplasm characterize some embryos. Impressive examples of normal development include the mid-bodies between blastomeres just after cell division, the smooth surface of endoplasmic reticulum and the dense arrays that form in it at 4-cell stages.

We come to the final stages of the book to cover the cleavage, morulae and blastocysts stages of development. Blastocyst formation as the inner cell mass and trophectoderm separate, and as the perivitelline space is formed, are highly significant features of early embryogenesis and the success of IVF. Examples are provided of degenerative characteristics in one or both of these tissues, which stresses how normal development and its detailed recognition is so essential for high rates of embryo implantation. Final stages of preimplantation growth include the hatching of blastocysts from their zona pellucidae. Examples of half- or fully hatched blastocysts demonstrate the beauty of these events. The final illustration shows paired protrusions from the trophoblast surface which may indicate cell division and a normal trophoblast. This is exactly the situation that is so important for the success of IVF therapies.

This book represents the realization of an immense achievement by its authors and designers. It must have taken constant effort and co-operation, a good eye for color, and immensely detailed electron microscopy. Its well-chosen micrographs and illustrations will attract many investigators and students of human conception. The combination of an up-to-date text with the detailed and relevant colored illustrations should also work hand-in-hand to create an easier understanding. It is also impressive to note that the authors maintained the pace of the text and the illustrations to the end. This has been no easy task, and my congratulations go out to the authors and assistants for their endeavors.

Robert G Edwards
Cambridge, UK
November 2005

Preface

For five decades, the images of cells and tissues produced by electron microscopy have offered views whose esthetic qualities cannot help but excite the imagination of both scientist and non-scientist alike. For the modern scientist, the ability to examine organization at the cellular and subcellular levels is an essential tool by which genetic and molecular defects can be related to normal and abnormal activities and processes. In our view, the long tradition of electron microscopy in the study of cell structure, function and behavior has been particularly informative when applied to reproduction, especially with the recent advent of *in vitro* fertilization (IVF) as a standard clinical treatment for certain types of infertility. Indeed, transmission and scanning electron microscopy has been particularly relevant in clinical IVF because it has provided fundamental insights into cellular and subcellular characteristics of gametes and embryos that are associated with developmental competence or failure. The aspects of female reproduction described in this Atlas were chosen because electron microscopy has contributed significantly to our current understanding of the normal and abnormal biology of human oogenesis, fertilization and early embryogenesis. The graphic technique of colored electron micrographs is used to depict different cells and their respective components because it enables cellular organization and architecture to be revealed in a manner that is both esthetically appealing and scientifically informative. For clinicians and scientists involved in assisted reproductive technologies, this format offers a unique approach to visualizing those tissues and cells targeted by protocols that manipulate or manage the menstrual cycle in infertility treatment. For clinical embryologists, the images of oocytes and early embryos may be of particular relevance in understanding the subcellular basis of certain light microscopic characteristics currently used to assess viability and competence. For patients undergoing infertility treatment, we hope that these images and the accompanying text can offer new perspectives into reproductive processes and an appreciation of the complexity of cellular events that, while largely unseen, contribute to or determine the success or failure of their treatment.

Sayoko Makabe, Tokyo
Jonathan Van Blerkom, Boulder
November 2005

Acknowledgments

Scientific collaboration:

Prof. Silvia Correr, Prof. Giuseppe Familiari,
Dr Tiziana Stallone, Dr Alessandra Camboni
(Department of Human Anatomy, Faculty of
Medicine, University of Rome 'La Sapienza', Rome,
Italy)

Prof. Guido Macchiarelli
(Department of Experimental Medicine, Faculty of
Medicine, University of L'Aquila, L'Aquila, Italy)

Prof. Jaime Pereda
(Department of Morphology, Faculty of Medical
Sciences, University of Santiago of Chile, Chile)

Dr Atsushi Tanaka
(St Mother Hospital, Kitakyushu, Japan)

Prof. Harumi Kubo, Prof. Goh Ohmura, Prof. Yuji Abe
(1st Department of Obstetrics and Gynecology,
Toho University School of Medicine,
Tokyo, Japan)

Dr Samuel Alexander
(Colorado Reproductive Endocrinology, Rose
Medical Center, Denver, Colorado)

Dr George Henry
(Reproductive Genetics Center, Denver, Colorado)

Mr Patrick Davis
(Department of Molecular, Cellular and
Developmental Biology, University of Colorado,
Boulder, Colorado)

Technical collaboration:

Mr Gianfranco Franchitto
(Department of Human Anatomy, Faculty of
Medicine, University of Rome 'La Sapienza', Rome,
Italy)

Mr Yoshiharu Mukai, Mr Hiroshi Fujita
(Department of Electron Microscopy, Toho
University School of Medicine, Tokyo, Japan)

Ms Toshie Shimozeki
(Department of Pathology, Toho University School
of Medicine, Tokyo, Japan)

Mr Tadashi Sakai
(Choubiken Institute, Tokyo, Japan)

Drawings:

Miss Francesca Brunone
(School for Anatomical Drawing, Department of
Human Anatomy, Faculty of Medicine, University
of Rome 'La Sapienza', Rome, Italy)

Artistic assistance:

Prof. Hiroaki Atsumi
(Tohoku University of
Art and Design, Yamagata, Japan)

SECTION ONE

The human ovary

HISTORICAL PERSPECTIVES

Since its first description by Aristotle more than 2000 years ago (fourth century BC), anatomists and physiologists have regarded the ovary with fascination as the organ in which the secrets concerning the beginning of life are hidden. Although various aspects of ovarian morphodynamics have intrigued investigators for centuries, the 17th century marks the beginning of key discoveries related to its structure and function. In fact, at this time, several scientists independently developed the idea that the human ovary was the site of egg formation. Renier de Graaf, in particular, was a pioneer in the field of reproductive biology. In the book *De mulierum organis generationi inservientibus tractatus novus* (1672) he gives the first description of ovarian (Graafian) follicles and the corpus luteum. However, his assumption that whole follicles were eggs was incorrect. In their early research on ovarian function (1666), Jan Swammerdam and Johannes van Horne, two noted anatomists, developed concepts similar to those of de Graaf. Another famous scientist of the 17th century, Marcello Malpighi, who is recognized as the 'father' of embryology and microscopic anatomy, was also fascinated by the structure and function of the genital organs. On the basis of his drawings and notes on the microscopic appearance of the cow ovary (1666), it was evident that he also observed what were later to become known as Graafian follicles. Malpighi called these structures *vesicles containing semen*, according to the common belief of that time that the ovaries were 'female testes'. It was Malpighi who invented the name 'corpus luteum' and who first described it as a gland, although he

could not appreciate that the corpus luteum was formed from the lining of the ruptured follicle. While his deductions were not always accurate, Malpighi was the first to provide deep insight into ovarian structure, thus outlining fundamental rules for modern microscopic approaches to the study of ovarian morphodynamics. It was not until 1827 when von Baer, on the basis of his own original microscopic observations, described for the first time with hand-painted illustrations that the mammalian egg exists within the follicle[1].

Many centuries after the discoveries and descriptions of de Graaf, Malpighi and von Baer, the microscope is still a wonderful tool that is essential in investigations of specific aspects of ovarian function. Indeed, as new submicroscopic techniques become available, morphologists and cell biologists in all areas of reproductive biology and medicine take advantage of these techniques in their research. This was true for transmission electron microscopy (TEM) and remains true with the most recent techniques in scanning electron microscopy (SEM)[2-9]. In fact, with the technological improvements of instruments that routinely use field emission, high-resolution SEM is complemented by sophisticated techniques of specimen preparation that allow highly dynamic views of the three-dimensional organization of reproductive tissues, cells and subcellular microtopographical domains.

The intent of this section is to present structural and ultrastructural aspects of ovarian dynamics that represent significant morphodynamic and morphophysiological events during ovarian development in the fetus, and ovarian function in the adult. Crucial pathophysiological events of interest to both basic scientists and clinicians are also emphasized, as this information should be considered when formulating definitive opinions about sampled ovarian tissue in clinical reproductive medicine.

NOTES ON METHODOLOGY

The images and accompanying interpretations in these chapters are derived from a large selection of human specimens obtained over many years of study. Ovarian biopsies were taken during laparoscopy or abdominal surgery in adult women[10-12]. Tissues from human embryos and fetuses (from the 3rd week until term of gestation) were derived from spontaneous abortions or surgical delivery (hysterectomy or hysterotomy)[1,13-22]. Gestational age was estimated through a comparison of several standard criteria including crown–heel and crown–rump measurements, the number of somites, and an evaluation

of the first day of the last maternal menstrual cycle, which should reflect the presumptive post-fertilization time. All human specimens were obtained with the patients' informed consent.

The sample fixation and preparation procedures used are relatively standard, and for light microscopy (LM) and electron microscopy, solutions containing 0.5–2.5% glutaraldehyde in phosphate or sodium cacodylate buffer (pH 7.4) were used[10,11,13-15]. The osmium–dimethylsulfoxide–osmium (ODO) method extracts the soluble cytoplasmic matrices from the freeze-cracked surface of cells[23], allowing direct visualization of the intracellular organization of both germ and somatic cells. In order to reveal fine details of the microtopography of ovarian tissues, connective tissue and/or extracellular matrices (including zona pellucida) were removed by controlled-timed osmium maceration[11,12] and all specimens were observed by field emission, high-resolution SEM.

1 Ovarian development during fetal life

The ovary is composed of two basic cell lines – the germ and the somatic cells – which differ in origin but are inexorably related to each other during the entire development and reproductive function of this organ[1,18-20]. The human germinal component originates from primordial germ cells (PGCs) that colonize the sexually undifferentiated gonadal primordium during the 5th week of post-fertilization development[17]. While the precursors of ovarian somatic cells are thought to arise from mesonephric tissues and cells derived from coelomic surface epithelium and mesenchyme, their respective contribution(s) is still debated[19,24]. Somatic and germ cell lines reciprocally influence each other during intrauterine life. In fact, the mechanisms controlling migration and settlement of PGCs in the developing ovary, and even their survival and differentiation, seem to be modulated by the surrounding somatic milieu[17]. Conversely, the presence of germ cells in the developing gonad primes both the sexual differentiation of the ovary and the onset of folliculogenesis. Endocrine factors, as well as substances with an autocrine/paracrine activity, are also involved in modulating gonadal growth[1].

THE PRIMORDIAL GERM CELLS: ORIGIN, MIGRATION AND SETTLEMENT

Origin and morphology of primordial germ cells

Primordial germ cells establish the germ-cell line in both the ovary and the testis. Studies and hypotheses related to their origin date to the late 19th century; Waldeyer proposed in 1870 that they continuously differentiate from the mesothelium covering the developing gonad (termed *germinal epithelium* for this reason). This hypothesis was in marked contrast to the findings of Weismann (1870), Nussbaum (1880) and Boveri (1899), who suggested that the germ cell lineage forms early in extragonadal sites followed by colonization of the developing ovary [for references, see reference 1]. These notions were confirmed several decades later when a remarkable series of findings was obtained in various species, including humans, using histochemical and other morphological approaches [for references, see reference 17]. Thus, as in other mammals, the life history of the human female germ cell begins very early and in areas that are not only distant from the developing gonad but actually extraembryonic in nature.

Despite the fundamental scientific interest in the origin of the germ cells that has extended through the centuries, it seems remarkable that where and when they actually separate from the somatic cell lineage remains unclear at the present time. Certainly, it occurs at the onset of embryo development and presumably no later than the peri-implantation stages, as shown in the mouse when epiblast cells microinjected into host blastocysts produce germ cells in the resulting chimeric embryos[1]. Definitive molecular markers for PGCs and their early progeny are essential for studies investigating the separation of the germ line in the early embryo. In this respect, a specific antibody labeling a PGC cytoplasmic epitope has recently been used for very early identification of PGCs in the rabbit[25]. However, similar markers for human PGCs have yet to be identified. The mechanisms by which PGCs are formed, how developmental totipotency is regulated, and the identification of factors that affect their development are some of the most important questions in modern developmental biology[26].

Apart from their origin, the earliest morphological evidence for PGCs in mammals is their detection in the endoderm of the dorsal wall of the yolk sac, near the developing allantois. In humans, this occurs during the 3rd week post-fertilization (Figures 1–3)[16,17]. By LM, it is possible to distinguish germ cells readily from surrounding somatic endodermal cells of the yolk sac, because the former appear larger and clear, and stain intensely for the enzyme alkaline phosphatase[17]. By TEM and SEM imaging (Figures 1, 4, 5), PGCs are generally round cells between 15 and 20 µm in diameter with well-defined outlines[1,16,17,19–21]. Their nucleus is large, eccentrically located, and composed of fine granular chromatin uniformly dispersed within a nucleoplasm containing one or two nucleoli. At this stage (3rd week post-fertilization), they display relatively few organelles with oval or rounded mitochondria containing tubulovesicular cristae, a single Golgi complex, membranes of the rough endoplasmic reticulum (RER), free ribosomes, polyribosomes and vesicles located primarily in the perinuclear cytoplasm[17,18]. The cytoskeletal system is relatively undeveloped with occasional microfilaments and microtubules detected, although centrioles are present. Glycogen particles and lipid droplets are common in human PGCs, particularly at the beginning of their migratory phase (Figure 6), and probably serve as energy reserves to support movement from the yolk sac to the genital ridge[18,19]. Focal contacts between PGCs and neighboring somatic cells (Figures 6, 7) involve desmosomes, intermediate and tight junctions. In addition, specific (communicating) gap junctions mediate germ–somatic cell interactions, although this type of junctional complex is not always readily distinguishable from tight junctions by TEM[17,18]. Taken together, these cellular specializations provide a structural basis for interaction between germ and somatic cells in which metabolic coupling may regulate developmental processes.

Migration of the primordial germ cells toward the gonadal primordium

The migration of PGCs to the developing gonad can be separated into passive and active phases. During the so-called passive phase, proliferating PGCs migrate from the yolk sac epithelium through the hindgut to the gonadal primordium[17]. The above ultrastructural characteristics are consistent with a relatively low level of metabolism that seems to support a passive hypothesis such that their initial transition from the yolk sac into the hindgut epithelium is a consequence of lateral folding of the embryo. It is at this stage of development that the embryo loses its discoid aspect and acquires a tubular shape, thus incorporating the yolk-sac endoderm into the posterior primitive intestine (Figures 2, 3). These morphogenetic rearrangements seem to enable PGCs to reach an intraembryonic position around the 4th week post-fertilization. At this time, numerous PGCs are found in the hindgut epithelium[18] and the active phase of PGC migration through the dorsal mesentery begins with their penetration into the underlying mesenchyme through small gaps in the basal lamina[17]. A comparatively small number of PGCs also reach the outer layers of the gut, although greater numbers are evident during the 5th week of embryo development in the dorsal mesentery that is composed of mesenchymal cells covered by a mesothelium (Figures 8–10). PGCs, often in small groups, are located beneath the mesothelial layer in close association with the somatic elements (Figure 8). At this stage, PGCs still show an intense staining for alkaline phosphatase[18].

PGCs exiting the hindgut epithelium temporarily lose their 'resting' characteristics, in that their former round shape and well-defined contours are now replaced by more irregular features including spindle shapes in which the long axis reaches 30 µm in length and the plasma membrane elaborates protrusions and pseudopodia (Figures 6, 11). Spatial remodeling of these cells is evident by a nuclear envelope that becomes somewhat irregular, and organelle movements resulting in their concentration in well-defined domains. RER membranes increase in number and delimit large intramembranous cisternae and microtubules, and microfilaments concentrate in cortical areas and within the cellular protrusions (Figure 11). These fine structural characteristics of human PGCs are shared by other mammals and are consistent with the acquisition of self-generated motile capacity. Accordingly, once they have passively reached an intraembryonic position, PGCs become capable of active migration by virtue of ameboid movements that persist up to the stage at which they reach the gonadal primordium. Thus, the amoeboid capability of PGCs demonstrated in *in vitro* culture studies and their structural characteristics observed by TEM are consistent with a fundamental morphodynamic capacity that probably occurs during normal development *in vivo*[17–20].

Although PGCs become motile cells, how they 'know' where to go during the active phase of migration is a fundamental question in gonadogenesis that generally considers two mechanisms: migration guided by chemotactic agents and migration guided by the substrate. For some vertebrates, PGC migration seems to be partially dependent on the production of chemotactic substances from the gonad-forming areas. However, how PGCs are chemically attracted to the gonad remains obscure. In the mouse, there is some evidence that a member of the transforming growth factor superfamily plays a role in such an attraction[27]. In addition, several molecules (e.g. integrins, specific types of oligosaccharides, E-cadherin) have been found to be expressed on the surface of migrating PGCs and to mediate PGC interactions with the surrounding milieu[28,29]. PGC specification also involves bone morphogenetic proteins 2, 4 and 8b, and the migration of these cells is facilitated by the c-*kit* receptor–ligand duet[30]. Experimental studies of PGCs' behavior *in vitro* and analyses of their movement *in vivo* suggest that their directed migration to the genital ridge is partially substrate-guided and involves specific components of the extracellular matrix such as fibronectin and laminin[18,29]. In this regard, a delicate fibrillar coat about 30 nm in thickness covers the free surface and pseudopodia of migrating human PGCs. This 'fuzzy' coat corresponds to a glycocalyx and is probably associated with binding sites for specific macromolecular components of the extracellular matrix, including fibronectin. Thus, this special PGC coat exerts a crucial role in adhesion to the substrate as well as in the recognition of the migratory route toward the gonadal primordium[1,19]. Other components of the extracellular matrix, such as glycosaminoglycans and proteoglycans, identified by histochemistry and ultracytochemistry have been reported to modulate or arrest PGC migration, as they usually occur in regions of the mouse and human embryo unrelated to gonad formation[31]. LM and TEM immunohistochemistry findings demonstrate that mouse migrating PGCs show immunoreactivity for the platelet endothelial cell adhesion molecule-1 (PECAM-1), a member of the immunoglobulin superfamily involved in vascular development and inflammation. This suggests a role for PECAM-1 in allowing cell-to-cell interactions through the migratory pathway of PGCs[32].

Although PGCs seem 'programmed' to find the gonad, some of these cells travel along misdirected pathways and reach ectopic positions. Most of these cells undergo degeneration but others can differentiate in ectopic locations as if they had colonized the gonads. It has been suggested that certain adult tumors (e.g. teratomas) result from the persistence of PGCs in ectopic sites. These germ cells, for reasons yet to be determined, exit a quiescent state and, owing to retained receptivity to growth factors and other stimulatory agents, begin to proliferate and differentiate in an uncontrolled manner. In some species apoptosis may have a biological role in avoiding the uncontrolled proliferation of these misplaced PGCs[1,13,19,33].

Primordial germ cells' settlement in the developing ovary

Between the end of the 5th week and beginning of the 6th week of human development, PGCs reach the gonadal primordium and colonize the most superficial areas of the developing ovary[18]. By LM they appear as large, rounded and pale cells intermingling with the somatic cells of the surface epithelium (Figure 12). By TEM and SEM, gonadal PGCs appear rounded or elliptical with small cytoplasmic processes irregularly distributed over their surface[1,14,17]. The occurrence of some gonadal PGCs with one or two amoeboid processes (Figures 13, 14) suggests a retained motile capability that may allow their continued migration through the ovarian tissue[13,14]. At the cellular level, the nucleus of gonadal PGCs remains large and eccentric, but the population of cytoplasmic glycogen granules and lipids detected previously in migrating PGCs is either absent or significantly reduced (Figure 13)[18], probably reflecting the exhaustion of these energy reserves that were used during the migratory phase. Small mitochondria, polyribosomes, endoplasmic reticulum and Golgi elements are by contrast well represented, and intense alkaline phosphatase activity is still detectable. Some PGCs, with a highly irregular shape, are occasionally found deep within the developing medulla[18], although their significance, if any, remains obscure. Failure of PGCs to survive or proliferate in the developing ovary can lead to infertility, while uncontrolled gonadal PGC proliferation may be associated with the development of ovarian teratomas or teratocarcinomas. In this regard, under certain conditions, mouse PGCs may give rise to a peculiar stem cell, the embryonal carcinoma cell[27,34].

THE DEVELOPING OVARY

The first morphological evidence of the future gonads occurs during the 4th week of human development with the appearance of two longitudinal prominences, the genital ridges, located between the developing mesonephros and the dorsal mesentery root (Figures 2, 3, 9, 10). These elongated prominences rapidly shorten and become hemispherical extrusions that bulge into the coelomic cavity. By week 5, the genital ridges are formed by different types of somatic cells, a proliferating coelomic epithelium that covers the developing gonad (the so-called surface epithelium, although at this stage the term 'modified mesothelium' is more appropriate) and an underlying compartment containing mesenchymal cells, blood vessels and mesonephric cells originating from mesonephric glomeruli and tubules that form the rete ovarii system. However, which components of the developing gonad have a primary role in the formation of the ovarian blastema remains unknown. After the arrival of PGCs, the gonad undergoes two main modifications: its somatic components undergo hyperplasia which increases gonadal size in concert with the rapid proliferation of PGCs; and the gonadal cortex differentiates and the medulla partially regresses when sexual differentiation in the ovary begins at week 7 (Figure 15)[1,13,17,18].

During week 7, organization emerges from what initially seems to be a chaotic intermingling of somatic and germ cells as cellular cord-like structures formed by somatic cells (the ovigerous sex cords) envelop groups of germ cells in cortical zones. These ovigerous cords are separated from the proliferating stroma by a basal lamina. In the areas in which the cords appear confluent with the surface epithelium, the basal lamina covering the cords is continuous with the underlying cells of the surface epithelium[13,15]. Ultimately, the primordial follicles arise by the fragmentation of these germ–somatic cell aggregates.

Germ cell differentiation: oogonia and oocytes

Beginning around the 9th week post-fertilization, proliferating PGCs initiate differentiation into oogonia. Although the oogonia generally appear similar to gonadal PGCs, they have higher mitotic activity (Figure 16). Oogonia possess a regular and smooth cellular profile and a scant cytoplasm containing a large, centrally located nucleus with little detectable chromatin and distinct reticular nucleoli. The cytoplasm appears 'pale' owing to the paucity of ribosomes and other organelles such as mitochondria (with tubulovesicular or plate-like peripheral cristae), Golgi and endoplasmic reticulum. Similar to the situation that prevails in gonadal PGCs, alkaline phosphatase activity is retained, but the residual complement of lipids and glycogen granules, if present, is further reduced from levels seen in these precursors[1,15,18,21,35]. The presence of an electron dense, granular substance, containing RNA and/or proteins, sometimes in close association with clusters of mitochondria, is often detected in the cytoplasm of oogonia. This substance has morphological characteristics that are very similar to the nucleolar material and has been variably termed nucleolar-like body, nucleolar granules, intermitochondrial substance or, most commonly, *nuage* (Figure 17). *Nuage* has been considered a cytoplasmic marker of earliest stages of differentiation of the germ-cell lineage in mammals[21,36,37]. Although the *nuage* is evident in male germ cells, it appears earlier in development in oogonia. A similar structure has also been observed in certain cells of the early rabbit embryoblast but its function, if any, at this stage remains speculative[38].

Oogonia tend to form nests of dividing cells that exhibit identical chromosomal configurations and are often joined by intercellular bridges (Figures 16, 18) to form a type of germ-cell syncytium that is thought to be a consequence of incomplete daughter cell separation during rapid mitotic divisions. The intercellular bridges are irregular cylindrical structures covered by a continuous plasma membrane (Figure 18) in which various organelles are sometimes detected[1,17,20]. These bridges and the resulting syncytium may coordinate differentiating and/or degenerative (apoptotic) processes that affect the germ cells within each nest. It has also been proposed that intercellular bridges could transfer functional organelles (primarily mitochondria) from germ cells that are destined for degeneration into 'privileged' germ cells that undergo further growth and differentiation[39].

Between weeks 12 and 13 post-fertilization, proliferating oogonia located in the inner cortex of the ovary begin to differentiate into definitive oocytes. As described for oogonia, nests of early oocytes are also joined by intercellular bridges. While meiosis begins at this developmental stage, it arrests at the first meiotic prophase (diplotene stage) and may remain in meiotic quiescence in women for 40 years or more. As development progresses toward the diplotene stage, the size of the oocyte increases and important nuclear alterations occur. During the leptotene phase of meiosis, the nucleus contains numerous fine electron-dense threads of chromatin and a compact, rounded nucleolus. Later, during zygotene and extending into the pachytene stage, chromatin threads undergo a process of shortening and thickening leading to the formation of chromosomes, paired and joined by synaptonemal complexes. The nucleolus is rarely observed in oocytes at the pachytene stage. While the nuclear envelope remains fairly intact during these stages (Figures 19–23), changes in the number and organization of cytoplasmic components take place. Mitochondria become more numerous and are arranged primarily along the nucleus with lamellar cristae oriented parallel to the nuclear membrane. The Golgi complex is also located near the nucleus and encircles the centriole (Figures 19–23). Membrane-bound dense bodies can be found in the cytoplasm. Typically, alkaline phosphatase activity disappears following the entry of the female germ cells into meiosis[1,18–21].

Germ–somatic cell interactions: the onset of folliculogenesis

Both nests of oogonia and oocytes are surrounded by a layer of irregular or flattened cells derived from the somatic cells of the ovigerous cords (Figure 18)[18]. These actively proliferating cells intermingle and enclose the germ cells forming rudimentary prefollicular structures often containing more than one germ cell. As development progresses, the 'prefollicular' cells continue to surround the oocytes when intercellular bridges are eliminated and fragmentation of the nests occurs. Presumably, these cells have an active role in the fragmentation process (Figure 24). True folliculogenesis in the human begins between weeks 16 and 20 with complete enclosure of oocytes by pre-follicular cells and fragmentation of the nests, and continues throughout gestation (Figures 25, 26)[14,18]. In these early follicles, desmosomes and small gap junctions are observed between oocytes and surrounding follicular cells and the oocyte–follicle cell complex is separated from the ovarian blastema by a basal lamina[1,18]. Somatic cells immediately outside the basal lamina are of mesenchymal origin and will form the future thecae folliculi.

The origin of mammalian follicular cells that will differentiate into granulosa cells during later stages of folliculogenesis has been controversial[24] since the 19th century, when Waldeyer (1870) proposed that the somatic cells of the sex cords arise from the mesonephros. This view is still held by many investigators and suggests that the wall of primitive follicles is directly derived from proliferating mesonephric cells that reach the gonad via the rete ovarii, located in the medulla-forming area, which then are segregated and 'dedifferentiate'. Other researchers have proposed that follicular cells originate solely from ingrowths of proliferating surface epithelial cells that penetrate the ovarian cortex and enclose the germ cells[13,15,17,18,40,41]. For the human, these different derivations may be irrelevant, as irregular fibroblast-like cells (similar to the rete cells) and voluminous epithelioid elements (similar to the surface epithelial cells) make up the wall of early follicles, suggesting that both surface epithelial and underlying mesonephric cells can play a role in follicular formation (Figure 25). The presence of numerous interstitial glandular cells in areas where primordial follicles form suggests that their secretory products may be involved in the early stages of folliculogenesis (Figure 27)[22], which results in the development of primordial follicles containing corresponding oocytes arrested in the diplotene stage of meiosis and surrounded by a layer of flattened follicular cells (Figure 26).

The reduction of germ cell numbers

Only a few hundred PCGs exit the yolk sac, yet this number rapidly increases by mitotic proliferation during migration to and settlement in the gonadal primordium. Oogonia, which originate from PGCs, not only differentiate into oocytes but also show a remarkable mitotic activity which results in their numerical expansion during the 5th month post-fertilization to between six and seven million cells. However, only a very small number of these cells (approximately 400) will ovulate during reproductive life, and follicular atresia and germ cell apoptosis have a significant role in the reduction of the pool of potential gametes during postnatal life[42]. On the other hand, the most significant reduction in human germ cell numbers occurs during prenatal development such that, before birth, the size of the germ cell pool is reduced to approximately one million[1]. In the prenatal ovary, two mechanisms seem to be responsible for the massive reduction in potential germ cell numbers: apoptotic cell death within the ovary; and germ cell extrusion from the ovarian surface.

Degeneration of germ cells on a massive scale begins during the 5th month post-fertilization and continues to birth. This process affects oogonia and, above all, primary oocytes in the zygotene and pachytene stages. The most common signs of apoptotic degeneration detected by TEM are swollen nuclei, alterations in the nuclear membrane geometry, condensation of chromosomes, mitochondrial damage, vacuolization and dilatation of endoplasmic reticulum membranes (Figures 28, 29). While the underlying causes of this massive cell death process may include genetic errors during chromosomal recombination and metabolic and/or vascular disturbances, degeneration seems also to extend to the surrounding follicular cells, leading to true follicular atresia[17–19]. Apoptotic cell death occurs in both fetal and adult ovaries, as indicated by the above fine structural characteristics, as well as by chromatin and cytoplasmic condensation, and organelle relocalization/compaction. The occurrence of membrane-bound particles in neighboring follicular cells or macrophages that presumably originate from the phagocytosis of fragmented oogonia are also indicative of an apoptotic process. DNA fragmentation, a characteristic biomolecular marker of apoptosis, has been shown to occur in germ cells by a variety of analytic techniques including application of the TUNEL assay to histological sections of human fetal ovaries[43].

The extrusion of germ cells through the surface of the gonad and their subsequent elimination in the coelomic cavity is another mechanism by which a reduction in the number of germ cells is accomplished prior to birth. This process has been studied in mouse and human[13–18,40], and seems to affect germ cells at almost all stages of prenatal ovarian development and, indeed, may continue during the period between birth and puberty (Figures 30, 31). Extruded oocytes are located in the most superficial areas of the ovary that are in close contact with cells of the (superficial) surface epithelium (Figures 30–34)[14,15]. Germ cells may actively reach these extrusion sites by virtue of retained ameboid

motility, or by passive mechanisms in which they are pushed to the surface as a result of morphogenetic rearrangements within the developing ovary. Once free on the ovarian surface, germ cells are presumably eliminated into the peritoneal cavity along with accompanying somatic cells. In fact, isolated and small groups of germ cells are common to certain areas of the ovarian surface during different stages of development up to birth (Figures 30, 31, 35). In other areas, rounded fissures are evident and are thought to result from transient perforations of the surface epithelium through which germ cells may be extruded (Figure 36)[14,15,17,18].

One interpretation of the above findings is that those germ cells eliminated into the coelomic cavity from the ovarian surface could be the same ones that had previously become isolated within the stroma and were transiently and loosely associated with the somatic cells. In later stages of development, when the sexual differentiation of the ovary into cortex and medulla takes place and the surface epithelium is separated from underlying tissues by a proper basal lamina, germ cells that had previously been associated with the most superficial areas of the ovary become incorporated into the surface epithelium and can ultimately be eliminated into the peritoneal cavity[13]. By contrast, germ cells located deep within the ovarian tissues and which were closely associated with the ovigerous cords during earlier stages of development maintain this relationship in the nests until primordial follicles are formed. These germ–somatic cell complexes (future follicles) are always surrounded by a basal lamina (Figure 37) and are likely to be those destined for further development or degeneration (follicular growth and/or atresia). However, even some of these may be extruded onto the surface of human ovaries at term (unpublished observations). In the human, formation of a continuous basal lamina that delineates both follicles and surface epithelium seems to be a critical event in determining the fate of the germ cells[14,15,17]. In contrast to the human, extrusion into the peritoneal cavity of healthy and degenerating mouse oocytes contained within primordial follicles is frequently observed during the perinatal period. In this species, oocyte loss is promoted by the fusion and subsequent disappearance of two distinct basal laminae: that underlying the superficial epithelium and that surrounding the follicle[19].

The long-held notion that a finite number of oocytes exists during reproductive life is a basic tenet of ovarian biology and one that distinguishes it from the biology of the testis, where a well-defined, self-renewing population of stem cells provides the billions of sperm produced over decades. The mechanisms of germ cell elimination and degeneration described above are the physiological bases for the massive reduction in potential germ cell numbers in pre- and postnatal life. The accumulated age-related decline in the number of follicles that can develop to ovulation (ovarian reserve) combined with normal loss by follicular atresia and ovulation become evident with the onset of menopause such that the occurrence of follicles at any stage of growth and development is rare in histological sections. However, recent experimental findings in the mouse suggest the possibility that germline stem cells exist postnatally and may be capable of oocyte renewal in the adult ovary[44]. If confirmed for the mouse, and if similar findings are obtained for other mammals including the human[45], one of the basic principles of ovarian biology will require revision. Moreover, the reproductive lifespan of women could be extended if clinically appropriate methods can be developed and applied to maintain, expand and control the development of putative germline stem cells *in vivo* or *in vitro*. This assumes that putative follicles that may be promoted to develop with germline stem cells in perimenopausal women or in premenopausal women of advanced reproductive age (e.g. ≥ 40 years) are able to grow, mature and ovulate competent oocytes. While this appears to be the case for the mouse under experimental conditions, age-related defects in human follicular biology that may render normal oocytes developmentally incompetent may also have to be addressed if the maintenance or restoration of fertility is to be realized (see Chapter 3).

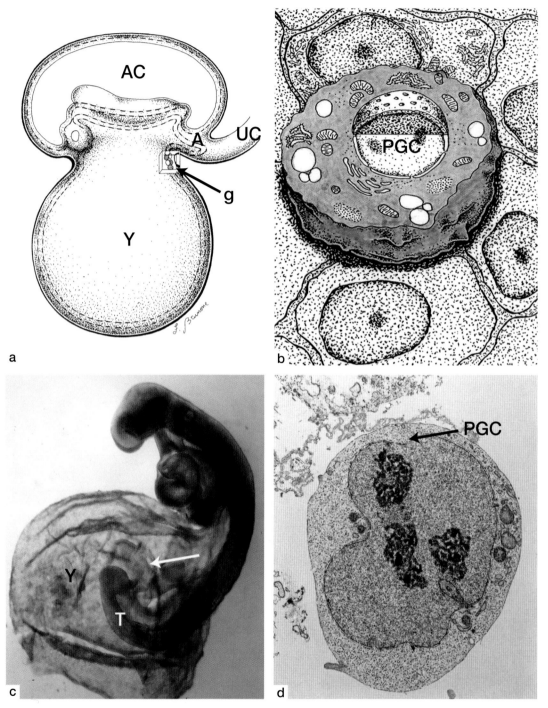

Figure 1 The earliest morphological evidence of the presence of primordial germ cells in mammals is in the endoderm of the dorsal wall of the yolk sac, near the developing allantois, which in the human occurs during week 3 post-fertilization. However, where and when germ cells actually separate from the somatic cell lineage is still a mystery; presumably this occurs very early in development, no later than the peri-implantation stages. (a) A diagrammatic representation of a lateral view of a 3-week-old human embryo, showing the position of primordial germ cells (g) in the wall of the yolk sac (Y), near the allantois (A). UC, future umbilical cord; AC, amniotic cavity. (b) A large primordial germ cell (PGC), 15–20 μm in diameter, is schematically represented among the smaller endodermal cells of the yolk sac wall. The typical primordial germ cell is round and contains cytoplasm characterized by the paucity of organelles. (c) A 3-week-old human embryo (18 somites). An arrow indicates the localization of the primordial germ cells in the wall of the yolk sac (Y). T, embryo tail. (d) A TEM image of a human primordial germ cell (PGC) located in the same region denoted by an arrow in (c), but in a 4-week-old embryo. The cytoplasm is pale with a few organelles. The nucleus has an oval contour and contains finely dispersed chromatin and three large and fully developed distinct nucleoli. The size, shape and ultrastructural features of primordial germ cells, together with their intense staining for alkaline phosphatase, make these cells easily distinguishable from somatic cells

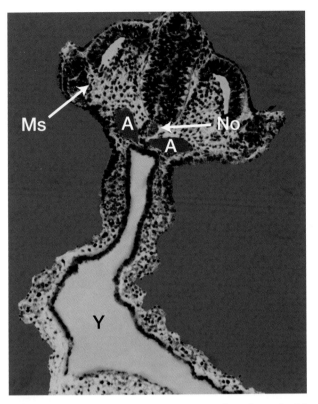

Figure 2 A transverse LM section of a 3-week-old human embryo in which the notochord (No) and the still duplicated aorta (A) are found in a central position, and glomeruli and tubules of the mesonephros (Ms) are seen on the lateral aspect. The yolk sac (Y), an extraembryonic tissue that plays a crucial role in the nutrition of the conceptus, is continuous with the primitive gut of the embryo. In mammals, primordial germ cells – i.e. the cells establishing the germ cell line both in the ovary and in the testis – are first detected in the endoderm of the yolk sac from which they migrate to colonize the gonadal primordium. Thus, the origin of primordial germ cells is not only extragonadal but also extraembryonic

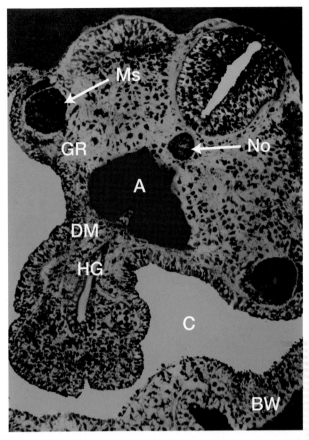

Figure 3 Illustration of the organization of a 27-day-old human embryo observed in LM transverse section. The aorta (A) appears as a single, large vessel located between the notochord (No) and the dorsal mesentery (DM) root at this stage of development, and the forming bilateral gonadal primordia are located between the mesonephros (Ms) and the dorsal mesentery. The developing gonads appear as two longitudinal prominences called genital ridges (GR) that protrude into the coelomic cavity (C). They are composed of a surface (coelomic) epithelium and an underlying compartment containing mesenchymal cells, blood vessels and cells originating from the rete ovarii on the neighboring mesonephros. Owing to lateral embryonic folding, the transformation of the discoid embryo into a tubular one results in the incorporation of a portion of the yolk sac into the hindgut (HG). As a consequence of these morphogenetic rearrangements, the primordial germ cells become intraembryonic and are passively translocated from the yolk sac to the hindgut. BW, body wall

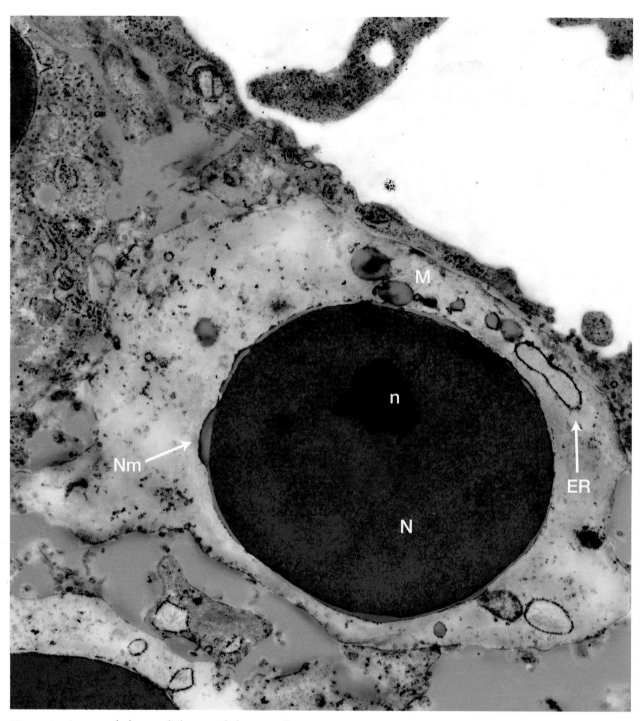

Figure 4 An irregularly rounded primordial germ cell as seen in the yolk sac endoderm of a 3-week-old human embryo, shown by TEM. The nucleus (N) is extremely large and contains a prominent reticular nucleolus (n). The nuclear membrane (Nm) is highly porous and the inner and outer compartments appear distended (arrow), suggesting active genesis of rough-surfaced endoplasmic reticulum (ER). The absence of a dense population of organelles is typical of these cells, and those commonly found in low numbers include mitochondria (M) with tubulo-vesicular cristae, a single Golgi complex, membranes of rough endoplasmic reticulum, free ribosomes, polyribosomes and occasional vesicles. This fine structure is consistent with a relatively 'quiescent' stage and tends to support the hypothesis that the initial translation of primordial germ cells from the yolk sac into the hindgut epithelium occurs passively

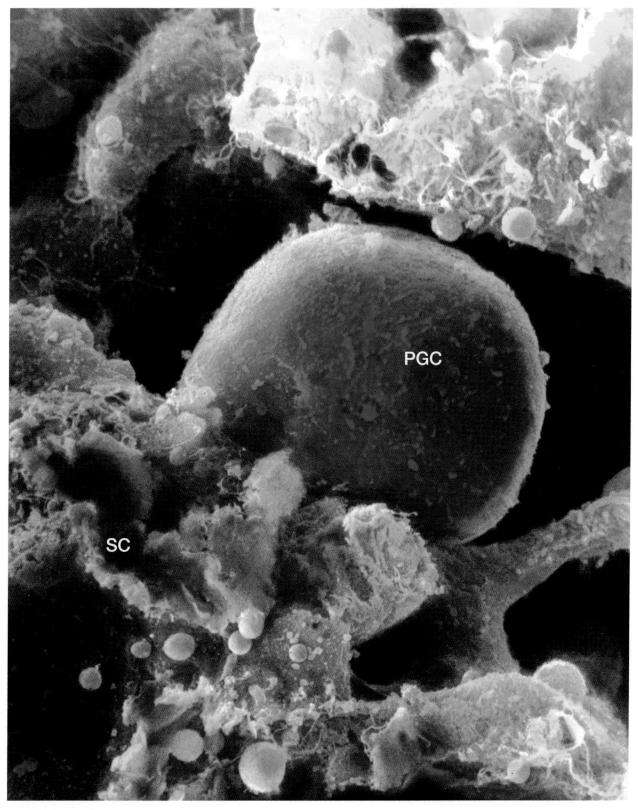

Figure 5   A large rounded cell (PGC) with a 'fuzzy' surface coat or glycocalyx as imaged by SEM is a consistent feature of primordial germ cells located between somatic cells (SC) in a 4-week-old human embryo

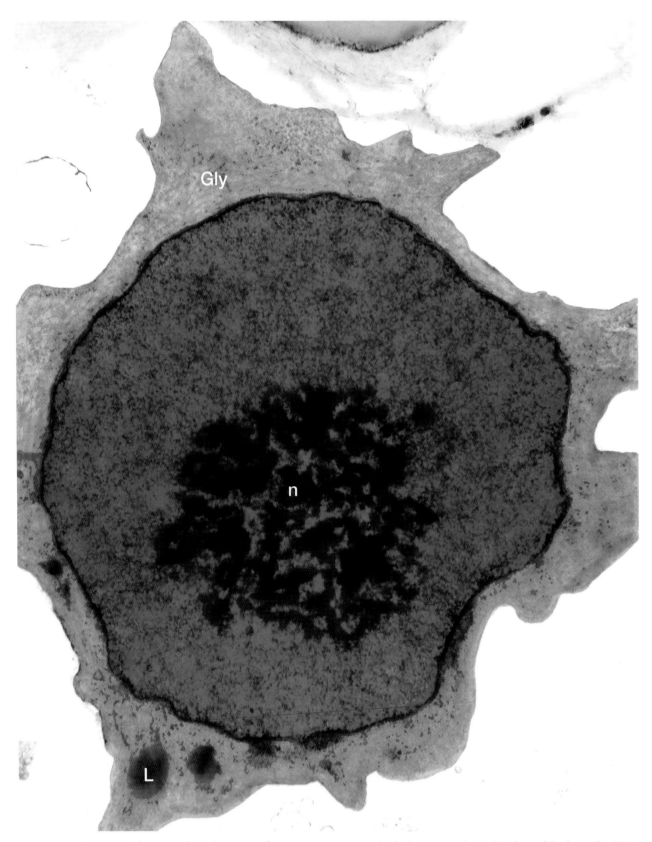

Figure 6 A primordial germ cell at the onset of migration in a 4-week-old human embryo (27 days old) shows by TEM an irregular profile that corresponds to the formation of numerous amoeboid processes that aid germ cells in their movement between somatic cells. The cytoplasm still appears sparse with respect to organelles, although glycogen (Gly) granules and lipid inclusions (L) used as energy sources are evident. A prominent reticular nucleolus (n) is seen in the nucleus

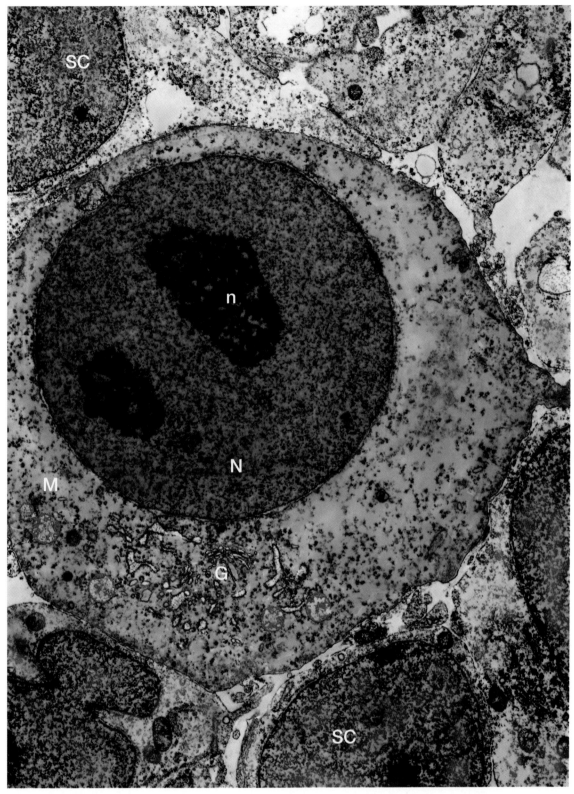

Figure 7 During the 5th week of human development, migration of primordial germ cells is well advanced with many of these cells associated with their somatic counterparts by means of focal close contacts involving desmosomes, intermediate junctions and tight junctions. The occurrence of gap junctions between germ and somatic cells is thought to permit metabolic coupling that may influence their development. In this TEM micrograph a primordial germ cell is found in contact with somatic cells (SC) of the dorsal mesentery in a 5-week-old human embryo. Most of the organelles, mainly mitochondria (M) and Golgi vesicles (G), are concentrated in a well-defined area of the cytoplasm. The nucleus (N) contains two distinct nucleoli (n) whose characteristics are consistent with high transcriptional activity

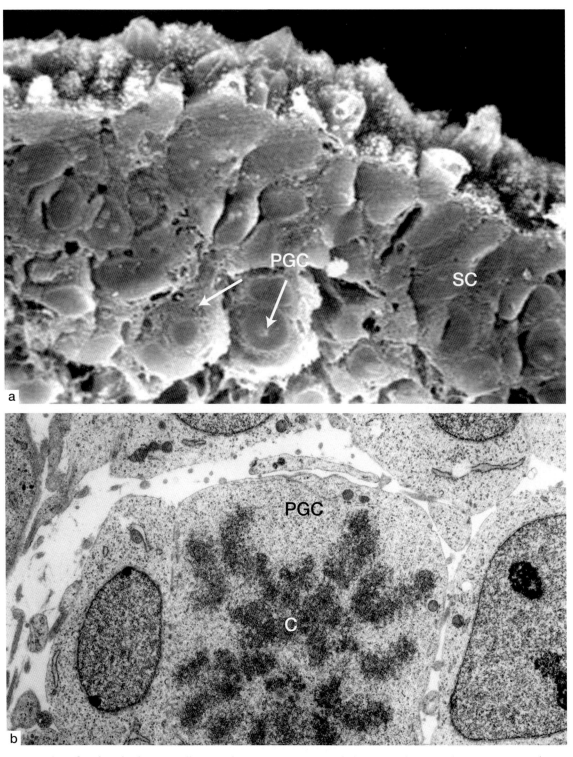

Figure 8 Only a few hundred germ cells start their migration toward the gonadal primordium. However, during their journey, they undergo repeated mitotic divisions that greatly increase their number by the time they reach the gonads. In fact, migrating germ cells are sometimes found clustered in small groups indicating derivation by successive mitoses from a single progenitor. In (a) and (b), migrating primordial germ cells are seen between somatic cells in a 5-week-old human embryo. One of the important benefits of sample fracture during preparation for SEM (a) is that it allows the intracellular organization of the primordial germ cells (PGC) and intercellular contacts with somatic cells (SC) to be imaged in three dimensions, thus offering a very close approximation of the situation that prevails *in vivo*. In (a), primordial germ cells are located between the somatic cells of the dorsal mesentery, a structure composed of mesenchymal cells covered by a mesothelium. The mitotic nature of these cells can be directly confirmed by TEM, as is shown in (b), where chromosomes (C) are observed to occupy the majority of the cytoplasm in a primordial germ cell (PGC)

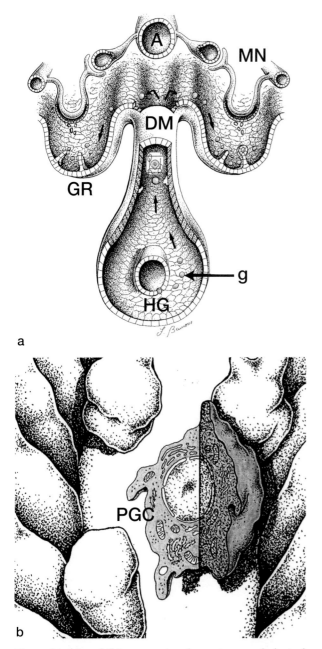

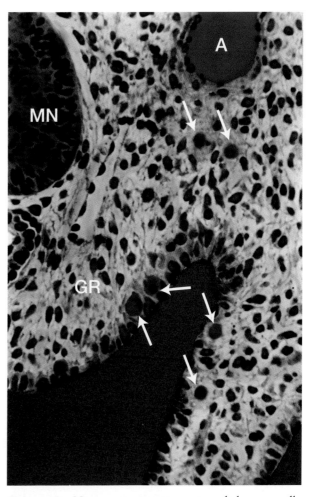

Figure 10 Numerous migrating primordial germ cells (arrows) can be seen in the dorsal mesentery and near the genital ridge (GR) in a transverse LM section of a 5-week-old human embryo. Portions of the neighboring mesonephros (MN) and dorsal aorta (A) are also seen. The development of pseudopodia parallels the acquisition of an amoeboid capacity during the last part of their active migration to the forming human gonads during weeks 5 and 6 of development. The directed migration of primordial germ cells may be modulated by two mechanisms representing short- and long-distance 'effectors': transient, focal cell-to-cell contacts and interaction between the glycocalyx and specific macromolecular components of the extracellular matrix over short distances; and chemotactic substances originating from the gonad-forming areas in the control of migration over longer distances

Figure 9 (a) and (b) summarize the major morphological changes that primordial germ cells undergo in the 4–6-week-old human embryo during the terminal stage of their migration to the gonadal primordium. The diagram in (a) illustrates the localization of primordial germ cells (g) in the early human embryo from the hindgut (HG), where they largely occur at week 4 post-fertilization; to the stage where they reach the dorsal mesentery (DM) at week 5; and finally incorporation into the genital ridge (GR) between weeks 5 and 6. The dorsal aorta, mesonephric glomeruli and tubules are denoted by A and MN, respectively. The boxed area in (a) is enlarged in (b) to show the most significant fine structural features of a primordial germ cell (PGC) moving through the dorsal mesentery. In particular, the previous 'quiescent' characteristics are replaced by an irregular profile with numerous cytoplasmic protrusions indicative of self-generated motility

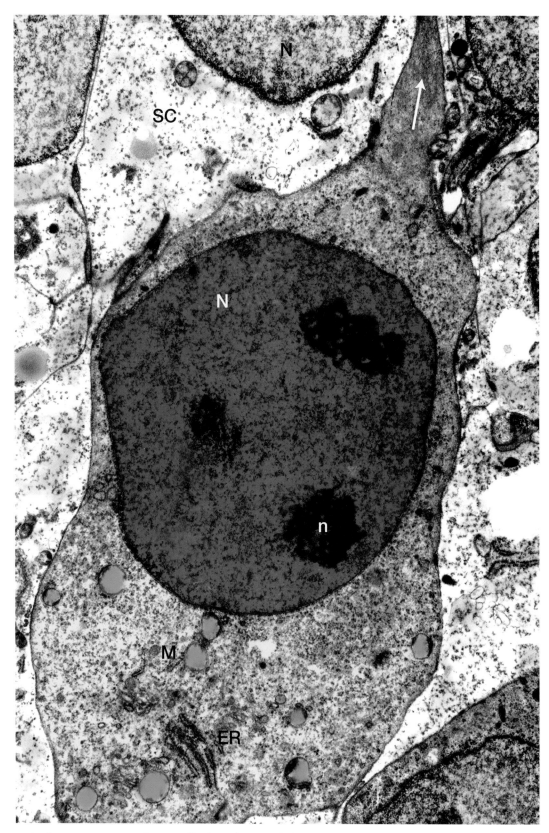

Figure 11   In this TEM micrograph a spindle-shaped primordial germ cell is found migrating among somatic cells (SC) of the dorsal mesentery during week 5 of development. The cell has acquired amoeboid features associated with migration and, in this section, a voluminous cellular protrusion (arrow) containing microfilaments is evident. Organelles, including cisternae of endoplasmic reticulum (ER) and mitochondria (M) are concentrated at the opposite pole. The largely rounded profile of the nucleus (N) is maintained during active motion. Well-developed nucleoli (n) are seen in the nucleoplasm

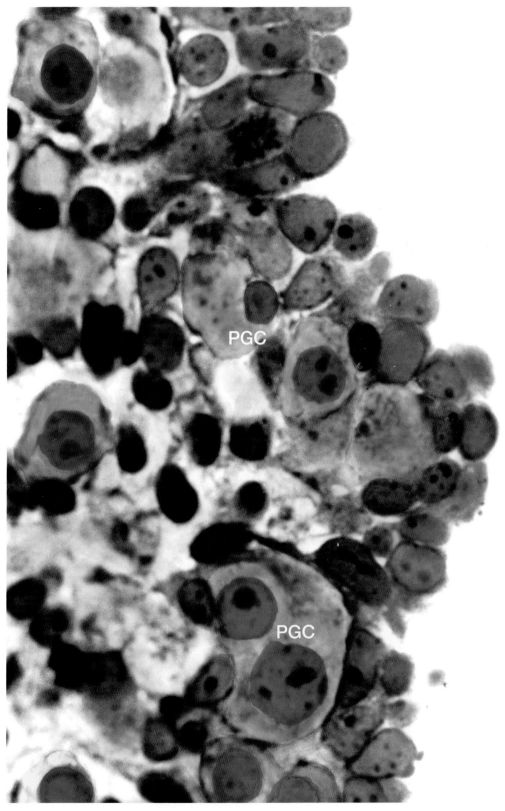

Figure 12 Between weeks 5 and 6 of human embryogenesis, primordial germ cells colonize the most superficial areas of the developing, albeit sexually undifferentiated, gonad(s). In this LM micrograph, taken from a 6–7-week-old embryo, primordial germ cells (PGC) are seen under the surface epithelium that covers the genital ridge. Germ cells, individually or in small clusters, intermingle with the cells of the ovarian blastema (surface epithelial, mesenchymal and neighboring mesonephric cells) that will assemble into the future definitive gonad. The presence of germ cells in the developing gonad primes both sexual differentiation and the onset of folliculogenesis in the female

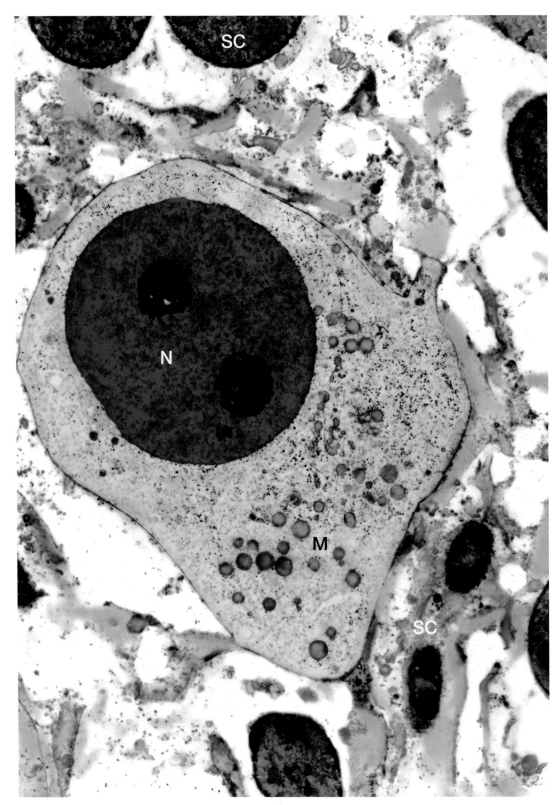

Figure 13 Gonadal primordial germ cells can retain a motile capability through at least the 8th week of human development, where they sporadically appear to be 'wandering' through the differentiating ovarian tissues. An example of such a cell is shown in this TEM image of a primordial germ cell that was found among somatic cells (SC) deep within the developing ovarian cortex of an 8-week-old human ovary. Unlike the cytoplasm in earlier stage primordial germ cells, numerous mitochondria (M), elements of endoplasmic reticulum and polyribosomes occur throughout the cytoplasm. However, glycogen particles and lipids are undetectable, having been used for energy production during early migratory phases. The nucleus (N) is round and eccentrically located

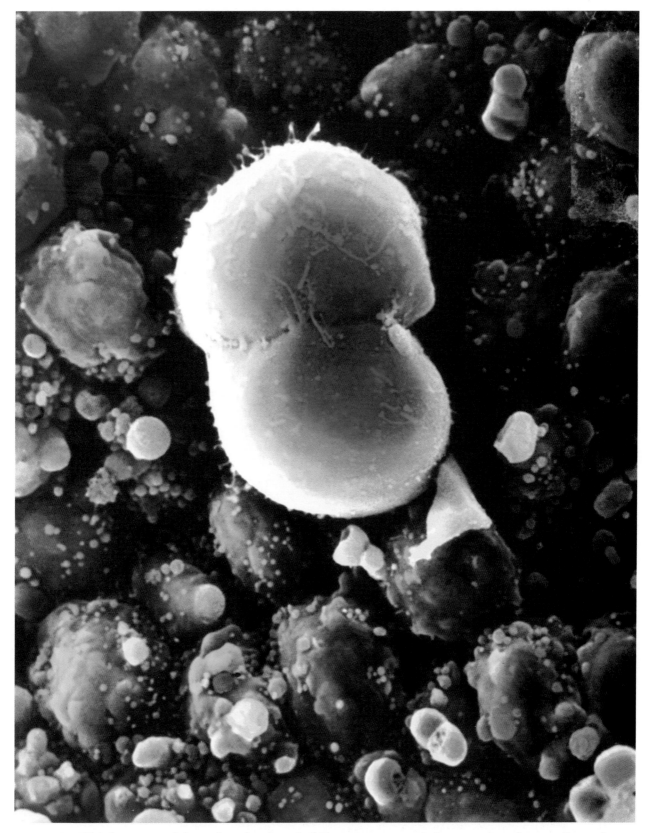

Figure 14   SEM observation of the surface of an 8-week-old human ovary reveals the occurrence of two small, round postmitotic germ cells still connected by intercellular bridges. After primordial germ cells reach the gonads, they continue to increase in number, as do the somatic cell components that also expand by rapid mitoses (hyperplasia)

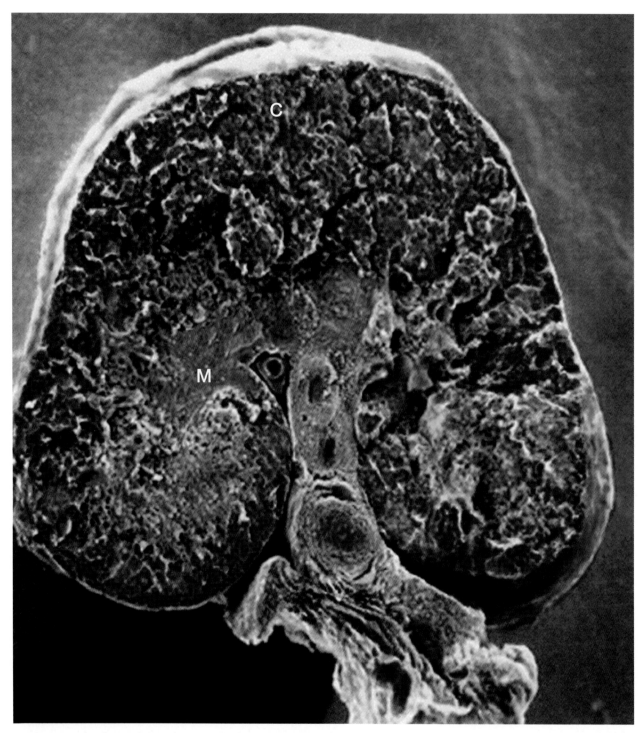

Figure 15 This figure depicts by SEM the fractured surface of a developing ovary in which the cortical (C) and medullar areas (M) have become clearly delineated in the 8–9-week-old human embryo. After the arrival of the primordial germ cells and with the initiation of female sexual differentiation during week 7 (post-fertilization), the gonad undergoes two significant modifications: somatic components become hyperplastic; and the gonadal cortex differentiates and the medulla partially regresses. In particular, the cortical area undergoes a process of condensation and as a result increases in both thickness and density. The inner core decondenses and separates into two compartments, the medulla and the rete ovarii, the latter of which is formed by reticular strands of cells that connect the ovarian blastema to the mesonephros

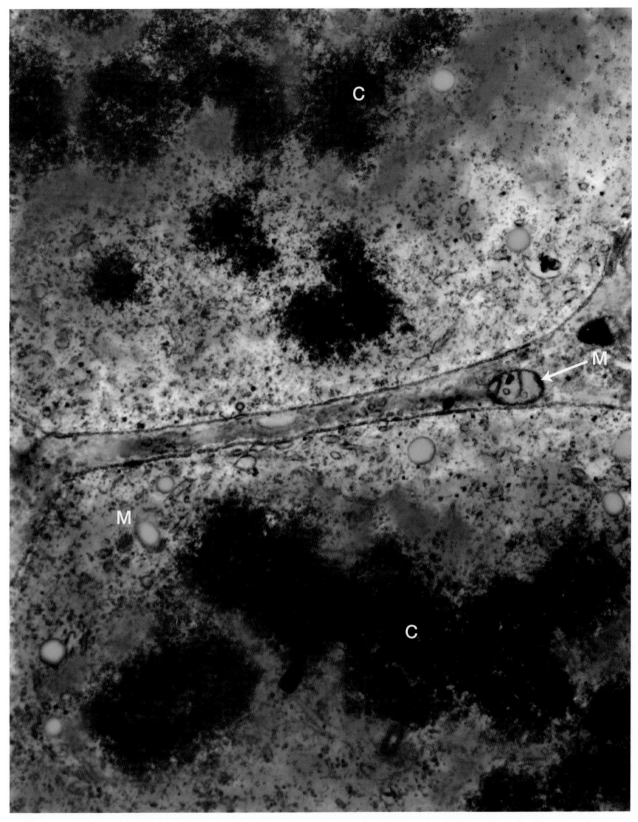

Figure 16 At week 9 post-fertilization, proliferating primordial germ cells begin to differentiate into oogonia, which are generally similar in appearance to gonadal primordial germ cells but have a higher frequency of mitotic division. In this TEM image, two dividing oogonia with similar chromosomal configurations (C) are seen in a 9–10-week-old human ovary. A few organelles, mostly mitochondria (M), can be found in the cytoplasm that is characterized by a scarcity of organelles

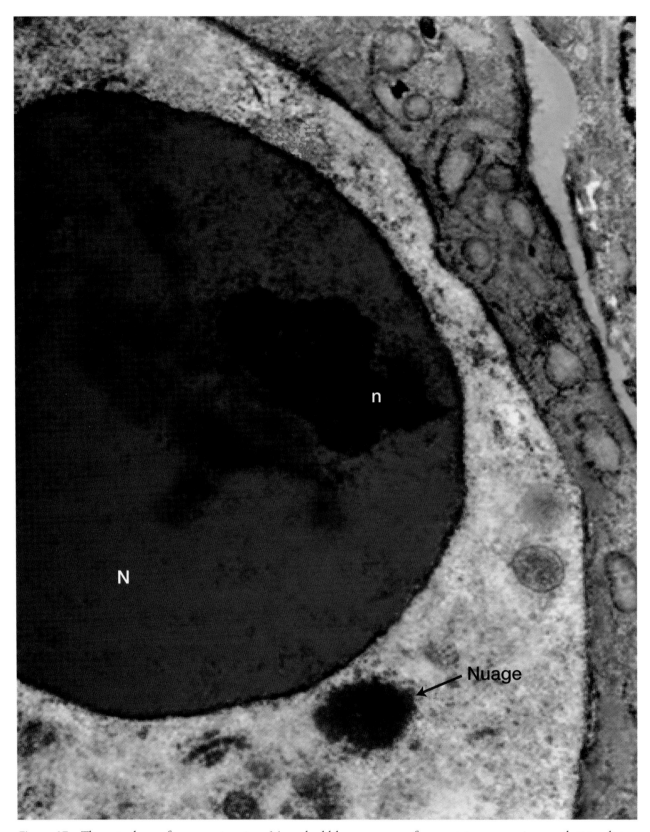

Figure 17 The cytoplasm of an oogonium in a 14-week-old human ovary often contains a conspicuous electron-dense, granular body (arrow) commonly termed *nuage*. This element occurs in both female and male germ cells and is morphologically very similar to the nucleolar material (n) inside the nucleus (N), and has been considered by some investigators to be a cytoplasmic marker of the earliest differentiation of the germ-cell lineage in mammals

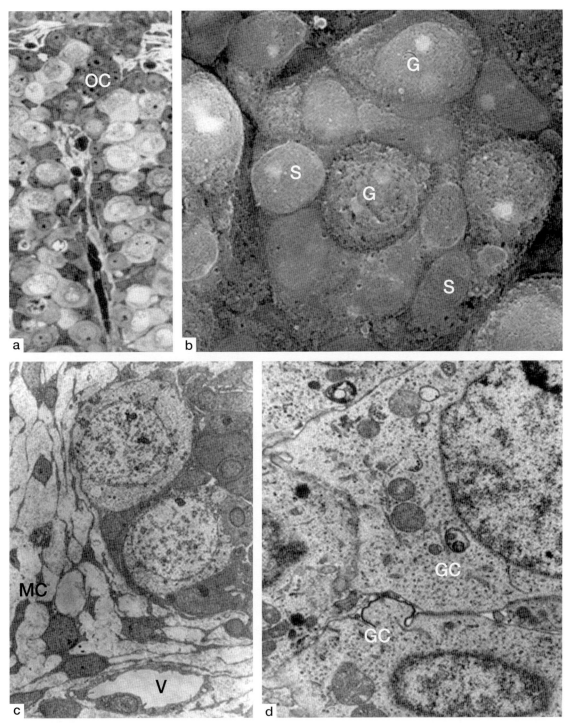

Figure 18 The development of the female gonad is initiated with and proceeds by intermingling of the embryonic somatic and the extraembryonic germ cells. Between weeks 10 and 12 of human development, proliferating mesenchymal stromal cells and vessels migrate from medullary areas toward the cortex. These fibrovascular ingrowths have a 'splitting' action that allows the formation of cord-like structures in the lower portion of the cortex that surround and ultimately enclose groups of germ cells. These complex germ–somatic cell aggregates become the tortuous and elongated structures of the ovigerous (sex) cords. The LM (a), SEM (b) and TEM (c, d) images in this figure are taken from 11–16-week-old human ovaries. (a) shows ovigerous cords (OC) in which somatic and germ cells closely intermingle. In (b) a nest of germ (G) and somatic (S) cells is evident. These nests are derived by the fragmentation of the ovigerous cords, and mesenchymal cells (MC). Vessels (V) occur in the interstitium between nests (c). Intercellular bridges that result from incomplete cell division during very rapid mitoses frequently form a syncytium-like network between germ cells within each nest. The intercellular bridges may coordinate further differentiation and/or degeneration of the germ cell line inside each nest. The two germ cells (GC) shown in (d) seem to be joined by an intercellular bridge in an 11-week-old human ovary

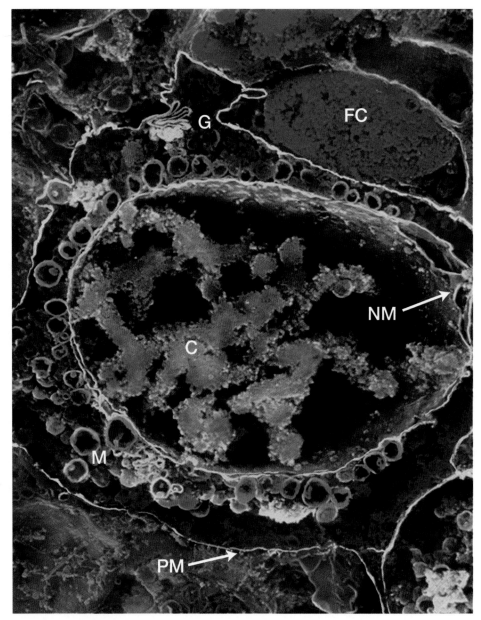

Figure 19 Beginning between weeks 12 and 13 of development, human oogonia located in the inner part of the ovigerous cords cease mitosis and begin to differentiate into oocytes. This process is accompanied by the onset of meiosis whereby oocytes enter prophase which is followed by the leptotene, zygotene and pachytene stages. Meiosis then arrests at the diplotene stage of the first meiotic division. Typically, human oocytes may remain meiotically quiescent at the diplotene stage (also termed 'dictyate' stage) for 40 years or more prior to their entrance into the growth and ovulatory pathways. Alkaline phosphatase activity, a biomarker of primordial germ cells and oogonia, is no longer detectable after the germ cells enter meiosis. Oocyte size increases and a conspicuous rearrangement of organelles occurs in the oocyte cytoplasm during the earliest phases of the meiotic process. Cytoplasmic remodeling mostly involves mitochondria, which increase in number as the oocyte approaches the diplotene stage and become largely localized in a perinuclear position. At the leptotene stage, the oocyte nucleus contains numerous fine electron-dense threads of chromatin associated with a compact and rounded nucleolus. Beginning at zygotene and continuing into the pachytene stage, chromatin threads undergo a process of shortening and thickening which leads to the formation of chromosomes, and the nucleolus disappears.

This figure is an SEM image of a pachytene-stage oocyte located between pre-follicular cells (FC) in the somatic cords of a 14-week-old ovary. The application of the ODO method extracts soluble cytoplasmic matrices from the freeze-cracked surface of the cells allowing high-resolution, three-dimensional views of organelles and their interactions with insoluble cytoplasmic elements. Here, numerous, rounded mitochondria (M) are seen around the oocyte nucleus which is enclosed by a distinct nuclear membrane (NM) and whose nucleoplasm is occupied by chromosomes (C) in the prophase (pachytene) configuration. A distinct plasma membrane (PM) surrounds the relatively small cytoplasm in which scattered Golgi complexes (G) are among the most evident features

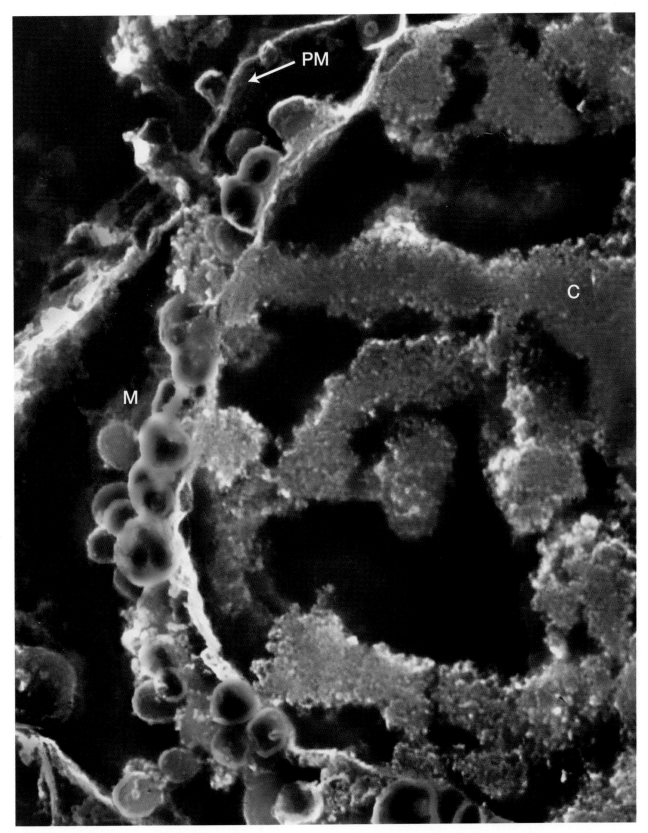

Figure 20 When Figure 19 is viewed at higher magnification, the direct association between mitochondria (M) and the outer nuclear envelope is apparent, as is the direct contact between chromosomes (C) and the inner aspect of the nuclear membrane. PM, plasma membrane

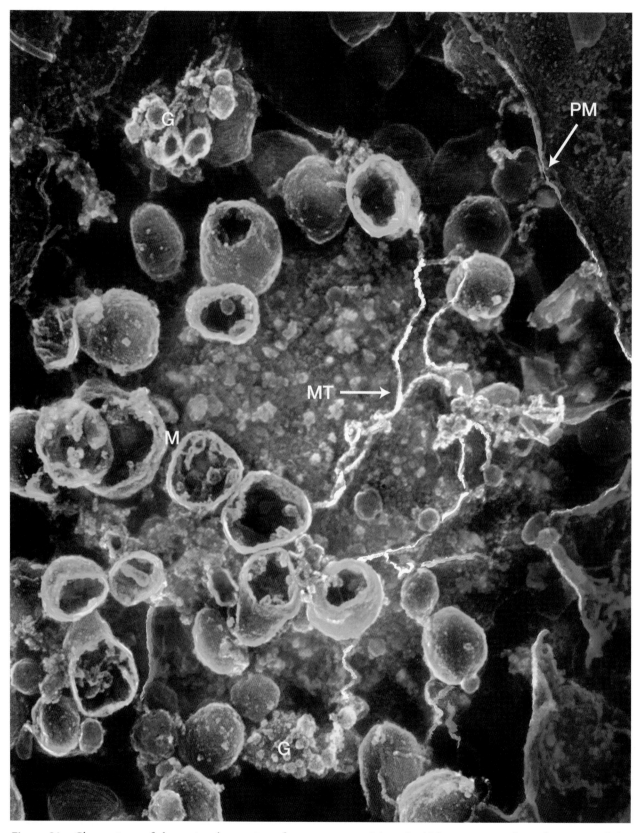

Figure 21 Closer views of the perinuclear region of an oocyte in a 14-week-old human ovary show that many of the mitochondria (M) gathered around the nucleus are associated with an extensive network of microtubules (MT). It is likely that spatial remodeling of mitochondria within the ooplasm is mediated by microtubules and that perinuclear clustering may provide higher ambient energy, which may be required for the progression of meiosis. Scattered Golgi complexes (G) are seen in the cytoplasm. PM, plasma membrane

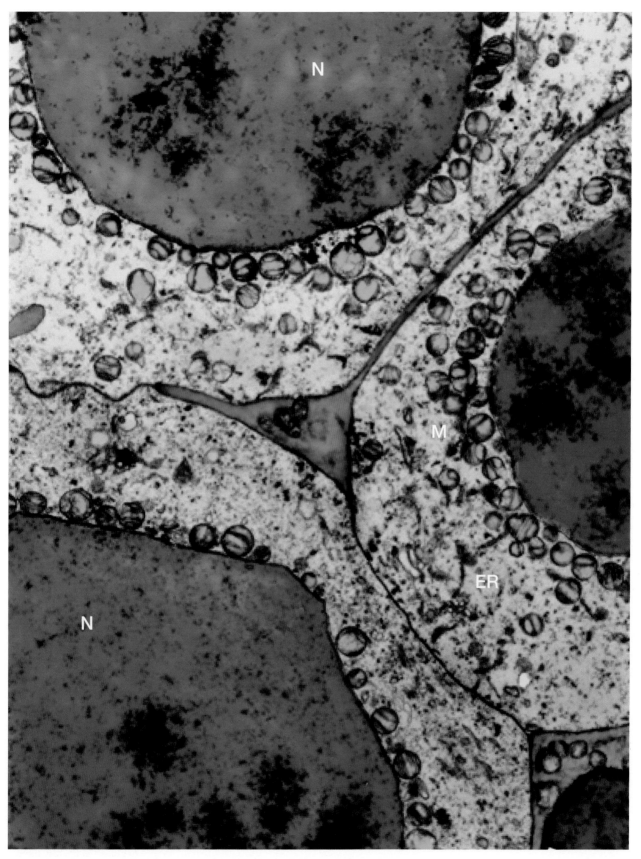

Figure 22 Three pachytene-stage oocytes still arranged in a nest are seen in this TEM image taken from an 18-week-old human ovary. Mitochondria (M) are spherical and disposed in a single or double row around the nuclei (N). Segments of the endoplasmic reticulum (ER) are a conspicuous feature of the cytoplasm at this time

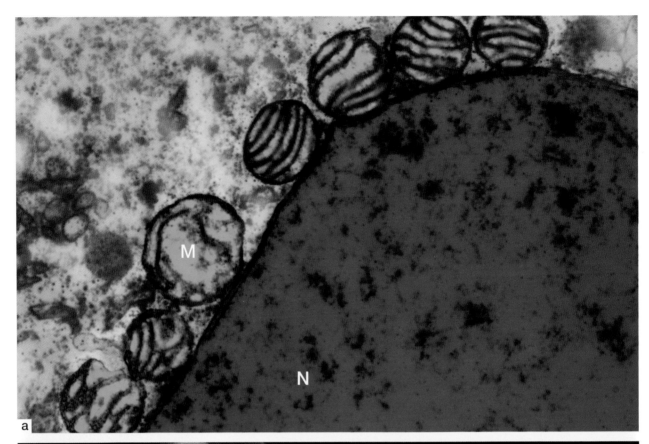

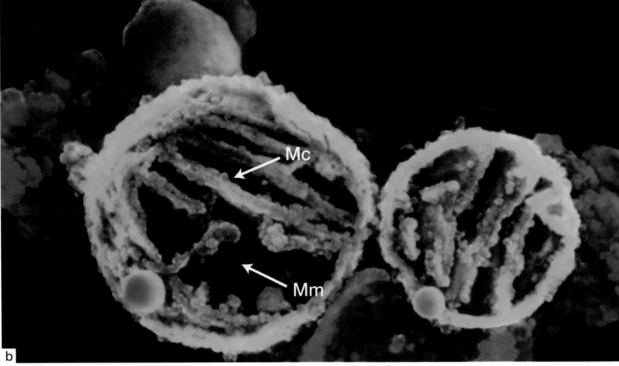

Figure 23 The ultrastructural characteristics of mitochondria (M) arranged along the nucleus (N) of oocytes at the pachytene (a) and zygotene (b) stage in an 18- and a 14-week-old human ovary, respectively. In contrast to their state of development in primordial germ cells and oogonia, mitochondria of early prophase oocytes have numerous lamellar cristae (Mc) that are oriented parallel to the nuclear membrane and traverse a well-defined matrix (Mm). This type of organization is typical of mitochondria actively engaged in ATP production

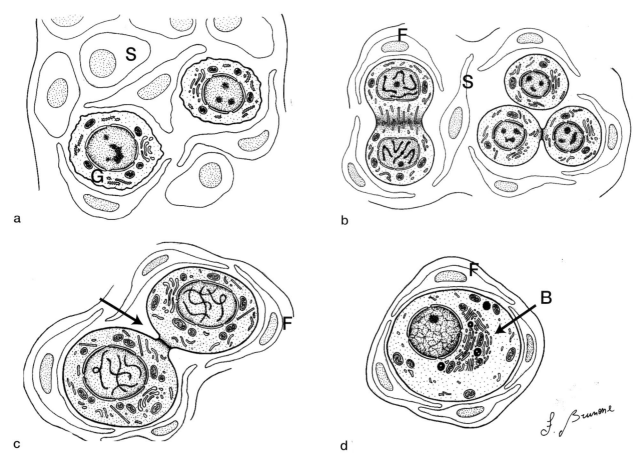

Figure 24 This diagram summarizes the morphodynamic events that occur during the early stages of folliculogenesis in the fetal human ovary, emphasizing the relationship between germ cells (G) and somatic cells (S) in the ovigerous cords. In (a), primordial germ cells are actively proliferating as they colonize the developing gonad. In (b), the mitotic activity of oogonia within nests is emphasized. In (c), an arrow indicates an intercellular bridge between two oocytes within a nest. In (d), a primordial follicle is formed by the fragmentation of the nest, and follicle cells (F) begin to surround the oocyte, whose most salient feature is a perinuclear collection of organelles termed Balbiani's vitelline body (B)

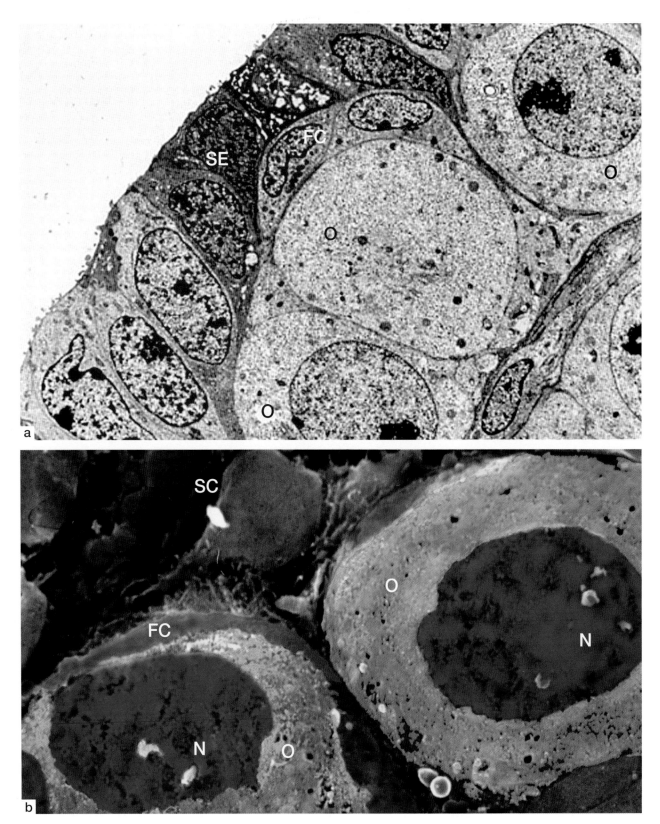

Figure 25 TEM (a) and SEM (b) images of a 14-week human ovary show the surface epithelium (SE) and surrounding 'pre-follicular' cells (FC) that originate from the somatic cells of the ovigerous sex cords (SC). The active proliferation of pre-follicular cells and their association with gonadal germ cells mediate the delineation and isolation of rudimentary follicular structures and contribute to the fragmentation of the nests and removal of intercellular bridges between oogonia. O, oocyte

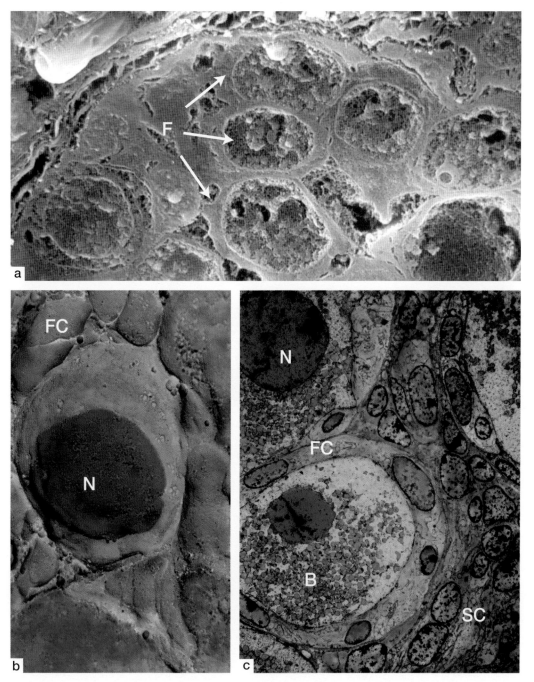

Figure 26 The earliest stages of folliculogenesis in humans are presented in these SEM (a, b) and TEM (c) images taken from 16–21-week-old human fetuses. Folliculogenesis begins during this time and continues to term. The onset of folliculogenesis largely occurs in areas that are extensively vascularized, presumably owing to more proximate access to nutrients and hormones. (a) shows ovigerous cords and groups of primordial follicles (F) in the ovarian cortex. In (b), somatic pre-follicular cells (FC) have aggregated around the oocyte, in which a prominent nucleus (N) is observed, from the neighboring ovarian blastema to form a primordial follicle. Several primordial follicles in (c) contain an oocyte surrounded by a single layer of flattened follicular cells (FC). These cells 'sit' upon a basal lamina and the follicles are separated by a highly cellular perifollicular stroma (SC). At this time the oocyte has grown considerably to approximately 50–70 μm in diameter and has reached the diplotene stage, where it may remain in a quiescent state for decades prior to resuming meiosis. In the ooplasm, organelles in high density are clustered at a pole of the nucleus (N) forming the so-called Balbiani's vitelline body (B) composed of mitochondria, annulate lamellae, Golgi vesicles and cisternae, membranes of endoplasmic reticulum, vacuoles, lipid droplets and lysosomes

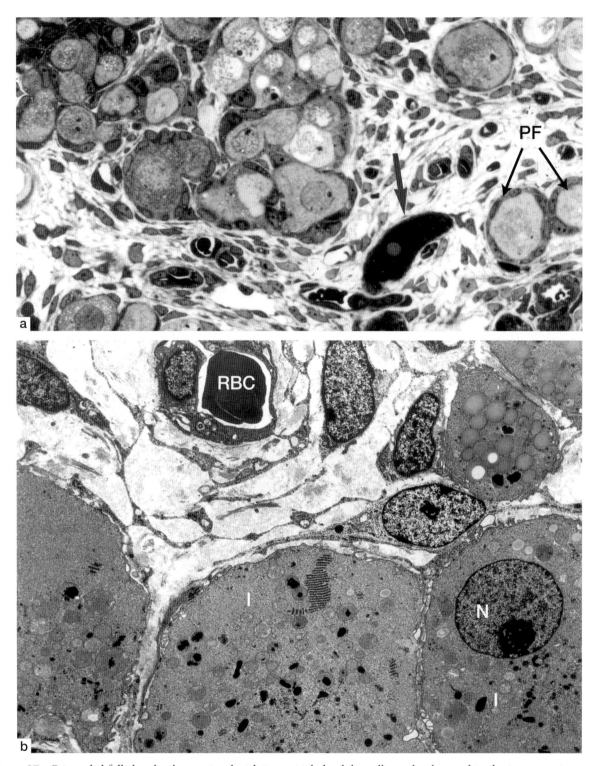

Figure 27 Primordial follicles closely associated with interstitial glandular cells can be detected in the inner ovarian cortex as early as week 16 post-fertilization. Interstitial glandular cells are particularly numerous between weeks 12 and 31 post-fertilization and have ultrastructural features characteristic of cells that produce and secrete steroids. It has been suggested that 'paracrine' activity relayed to steroid production by interstitial glandular cells may mediate the development of the ovigerous cords, their fragmentation into nests, and subsequent evolution into primordial follicles. In (a) (LM micrograph), several primordial follicles (PF) occur in proximity to a single prominent interstitial glandular cell (arrow) contained within a loose connective tissue composed of fibrocytes and blood vessels located within the deepest ingrowths of the ovigerous cords. In (b) (TEM micrograph), a cluster of interstitial glandular cells (I) partially surrounded by fibrocytes is observed in proximity to a red blood cell (RBC)-containing capillary vessel that courses though a mesh-like scaffold formed by fibrocytes. The nucleus (N) of an interstitial glandular cell is also seen. Both images were taken from a 16-week-old human ovary

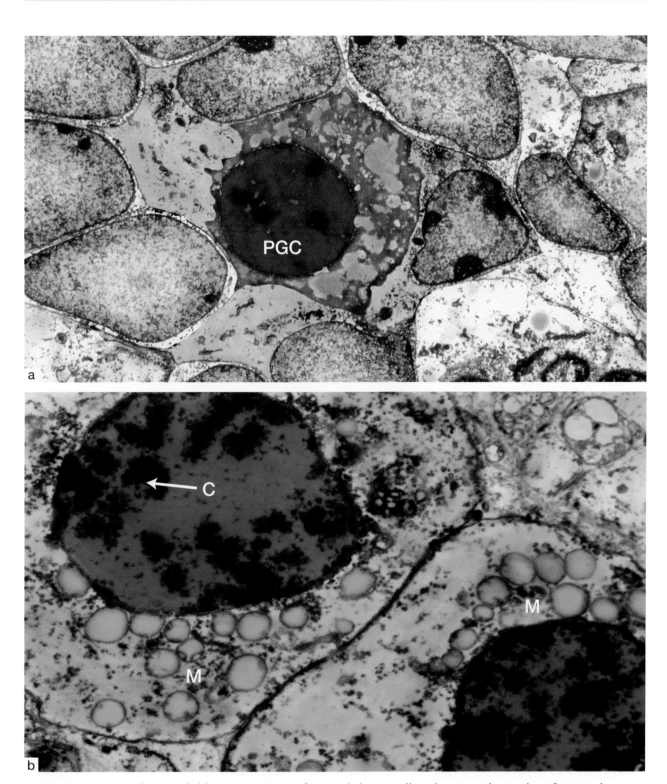

Figure 28 Owing to the remarkable mitotic activity of primordial germ cells and oogonia, the number of potential oocytes in a fetal human ovary reaches a peak of about 6–7 million during the fifth month of development. However, a massive decrease in germ cell number occurs in the prenatal period such that approximately 2 million oocytes occur in both ovaries at birth, of which nearly half show signs of degeneration. This reduction in the number of potential oocytes occurs at all stages of oogenesis, including the primordial germ cell phase. In (a), a degenerating primordial germ cell (PGC) is seen by TEM during its migration in a 4-week-old human embryo, and in (b) two degenerating germ cells are observable in a 14-week-old human ovary. In both the fetal and adult ovary, programmed cell death by apoptosis is the primary mechanism responsible for this regressive phenomenon. The condensation of chromatin (C) within the nucleus and the loss of cristae in swollen mitochondria (M) are degenerative nuclear and cytoplasmic changes characteristic of apoptosis

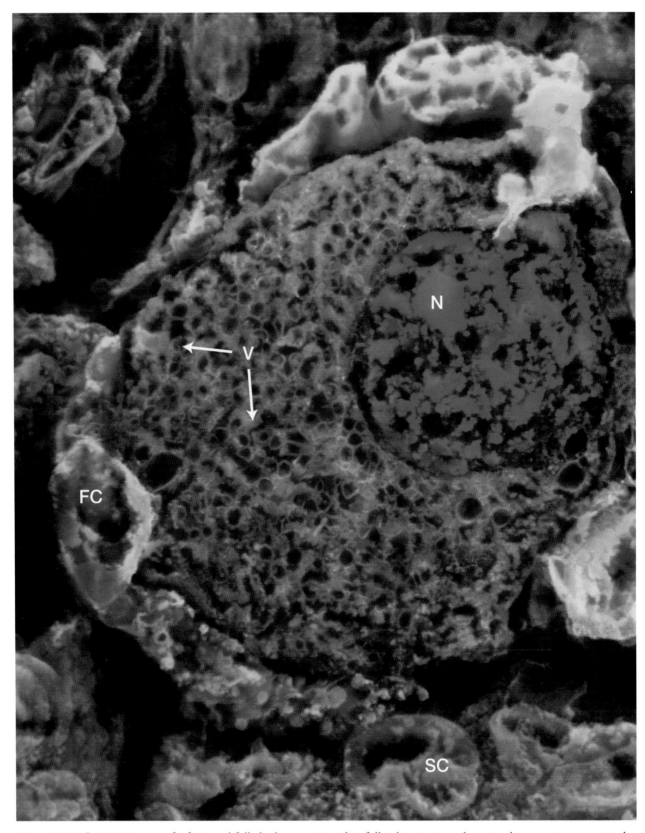

Figure 29 This SEM image of a fractured follicle demonstrates that follicular atresia and oocyte degeneration occur in the term human ovary. The follicle cells (FC) are irregular in shape and, in some that are highly flattened, the presence of surface blebs and indentations is indicative of apoptosis. Likewise, the oocyte cytoplasm is extensively vacuolated (V) and the nuclear matrix (N) is condensed, which are signs of a premorbid condition. SC, stromal cells of the interstitium

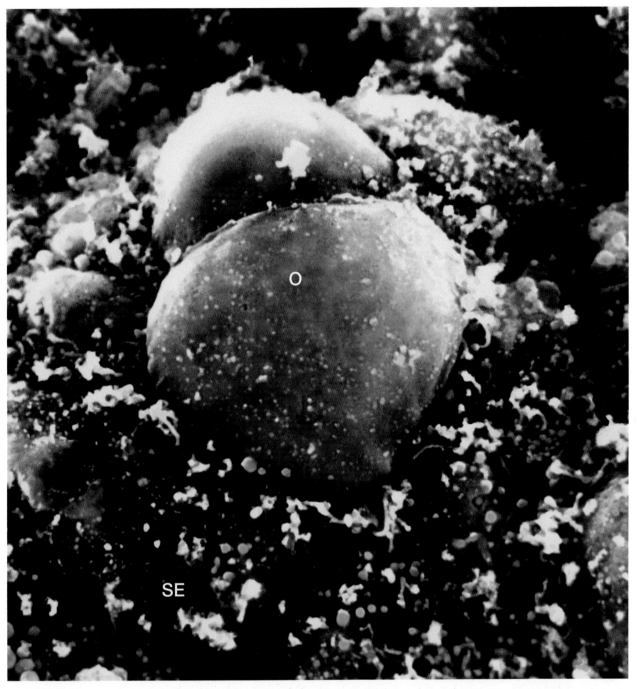

Figure 30 In addition to apoptosis, the physical expulsion of germ cells (oogonia and oocytes) from the developing ovary is another mechanism by which the number of oocytes may be substantially reduced during the prenatal development of the human female. In this SEM image taken from an 18-week-old human ovary, two oogonia (O) have been extruded onto the ovarian superficial epithelium (SE), where they will ultimately be eliminated into the celomic cavity

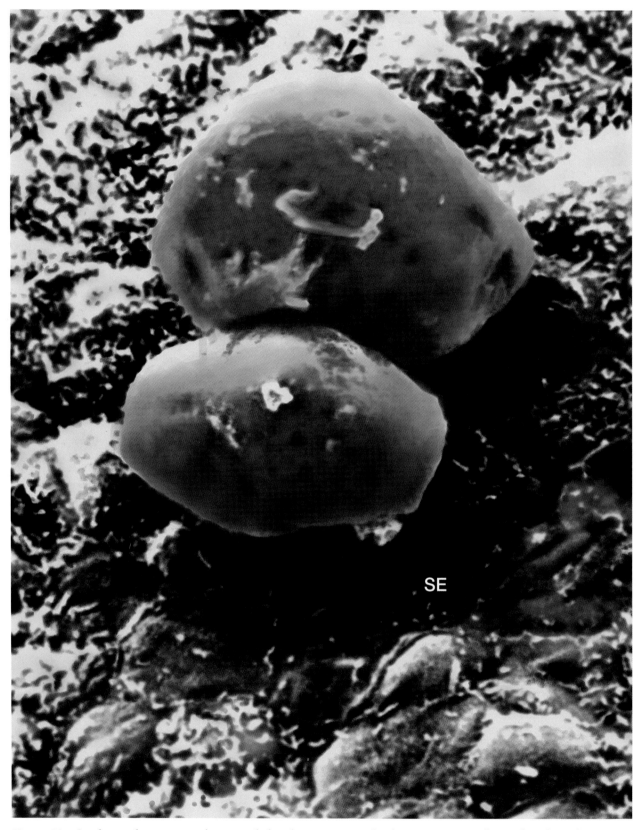

Figure 31 Similar to the situation that prevailed earlier in ovarian development, germ cells are found on the ovarian surface at term. In this SEM image, two oocytes devoid of their follicle cell component are seen on the surface of the ovarian superficial epithelium (SE)

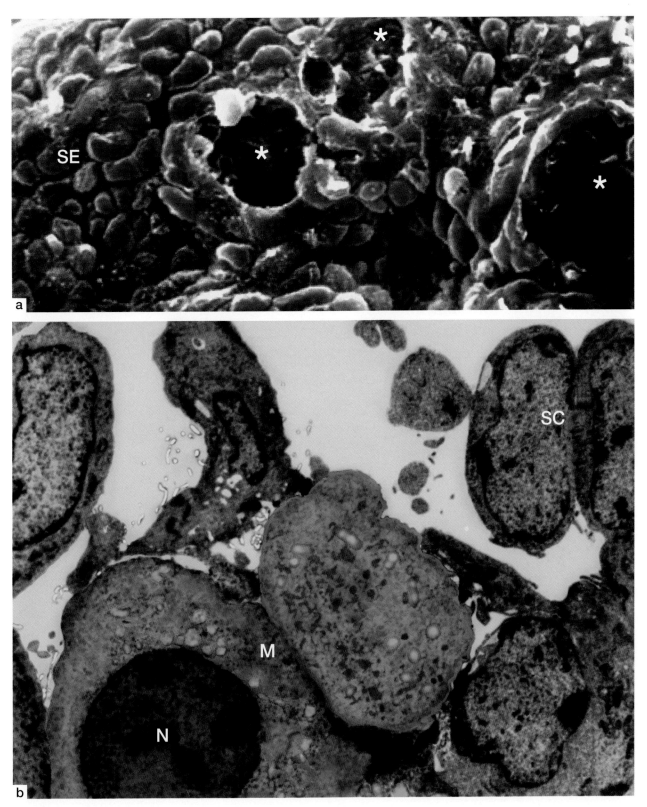

Figure 32 The process by which germ cells may be physically expelled from the developing ovary is seen in these SEM (a) and TEM (b) images taken from a 20–21-week-old human ovary. The surface epithelial cells appear to be exfoliating into the peritoneal cavity forming crypt-like structures (asterisks, a) through which germ cells emerge onto the ovarian surface. Germ cells may reach these sites during early developmental stages when they still retain ameboid movements or may be passively eliminated during more advanced stages owing to underlying morphogenetic rearrangements. Two germ cells on the surface of the developing ovary are shown in cross section in (b), where they appear to be located between disrupted superficial cells (SC). Numerous mitochondria (M) populate the germ cell cytoplasm. N, nucleus of a germ cell

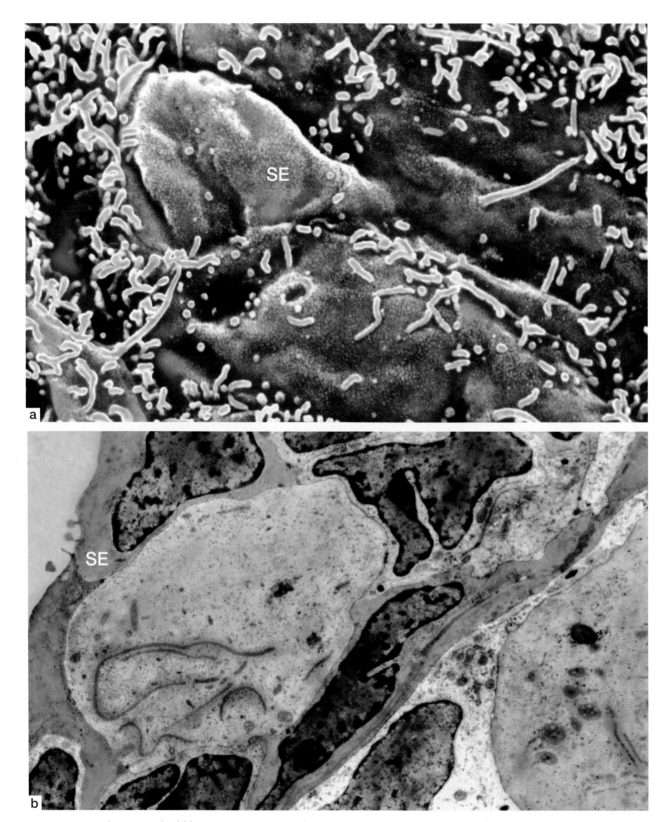

Figure 33 In the 24-week-old human ovary, SEM analysis shows numerous regions of surface epithelial cells (SE) that are highly flattened, most likely as a consequence of pressure from subjacent germ cells (a) and, when examined by TEM (b), the germ cells are completely enclosed by the surface epithelial layer. These images are consistent with a mechanism of germ cell extrusion onto the ovarian surface and subsequent elimination into the coelomic cavity

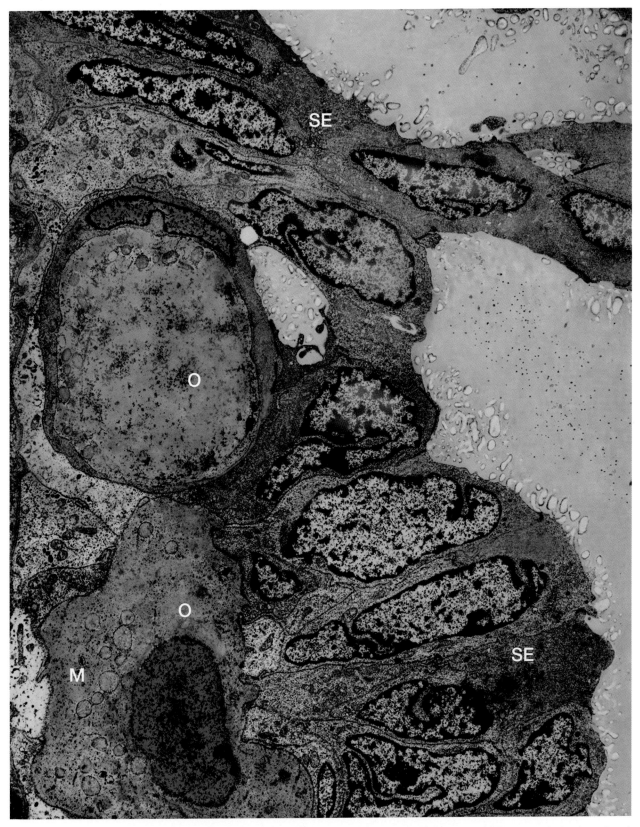

Figure 34   In the term ovary, the cylindrical or cuboidal cells of the superficial epithelium (SE) are regularly aligned and associated with an underlying basal lamina. Their nuclei have a characteristic oval or indented appearance and contain uniformly dispersed chromatin and peripheral patches of heterochromatin. In this TEM image, two oocytes (O) are in close proximity to the superficial epithelium and may be in a pre-expulsion location. M, oocyte mitochondria

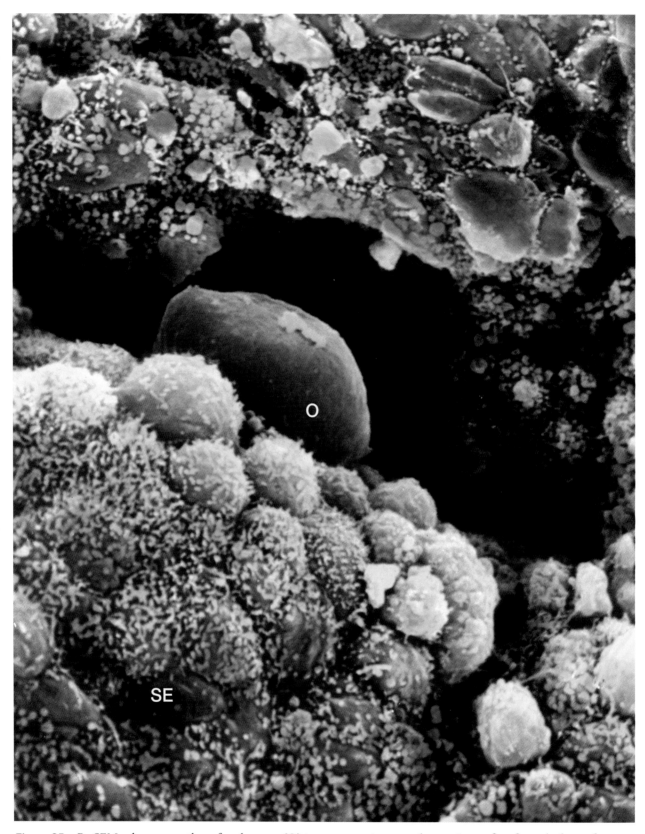

Figure 35 By SEM, a large, smooth-surfaced oocyte (O) is seen emerging onto the ovarian surface from the base of a crypt contained within the superficial epithelium (SE) of a term human ovary

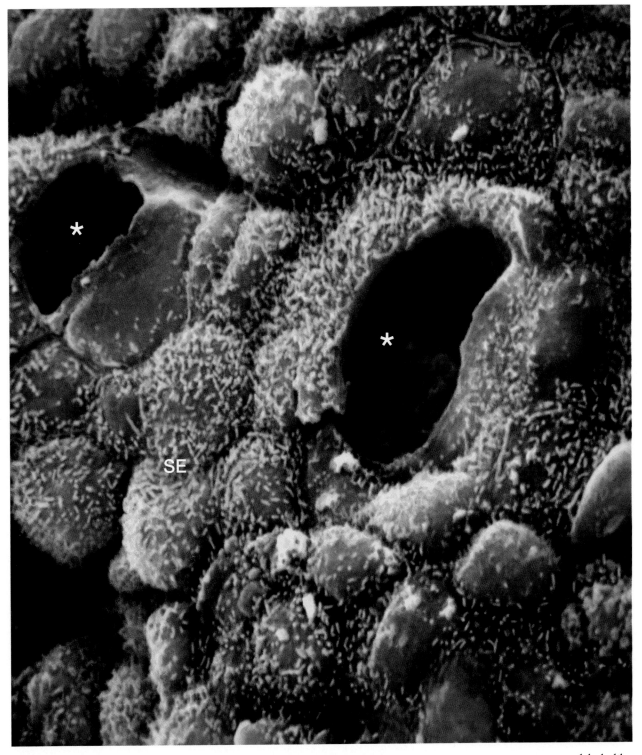

Figure 36 In this high-magnification SEM view of the surface of a human ovary at term, numerous round hole-like structures (asterisks) are observed. These formations are thought to be temporary openings in the superficial epithelium (SE) through which oocytes have been extruded onto the ovarian surface

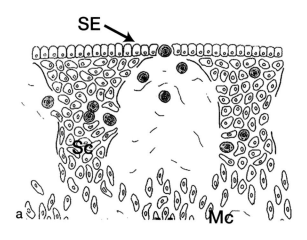

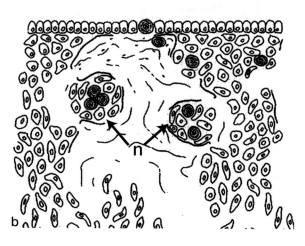

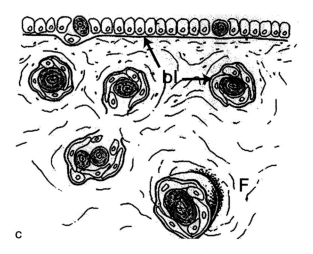

Figure 37 This drawing summarizes the two fates of germ cells in the developing human ovary: elimination from the ovarian surface or enclosure within early follicles as they relate to the formation of a basal lamina. When ovigerous cords begin to form they become separated from the proliferating stroma by a basal lamina. In the areas where the cords appear confluent with the superficial epithelium, the basal lamina covering the cords extends to the underlying surface of epithelial cells. Later, when the ovigerous cords undergo fragmentation and the surface epithelium become underlined by a proper, continuous basal lamina, germ cells that had previously been associated with the outermost areas of the ovary become incorporated into the superficial epithelium and then eliminated into the peritoneal cavity. By contrast, germ cells that in earlier developmental stages were located deep within the cortex and enclosed within the ovigerous cords maintain this relationship up to the development of primordial follicles. Each follicle becomes surrounded by an individual basal lamina that originates from the cords. In the human, the formation of a basal lamina delimits the surface epithelium on one side and the ovarian follicles on the other and this may be an important event in folliculogenesis and one that allows the fate of germ cells to be followed for analytical purposes. (a) shows the proliferation of ovigerous cords from both somatic cells (Sc) and mesonephric cells (Mc) below a superficial epithelium (SE). In (b), nests (n) containing more than one germ cell have segregated within the ovigerous cords. (c) illustrates the formation of a continuous basal lamina (bl) beneath the superficial epithelium and around the primordial follicles (F) that develop by fragmentation of pre-existing nests

2   The adult human ovary

The ovaries are paired organs responsible for the production of the female gametes, termed ova or oocytes, and for the secretion of two essential endocrine sex hormones, estrogen and progesterone. Similar to its male counterpart the testis, the ovary is a unique organ that contains both germ cells and somatic 'nurse' cells, the granulosa or follicle cells, which co-organize with the oocyte to form the basic unit of the ovary, the follicle. The somatic cell component has often been considered a specialized adult stem cell owing to its capacity to proliferate, self-renew and generate differentiated progeny with distinctly different functions. Some of these cells have a regenerative capacity, which is especially evident after injury associated with ovulation, and the ability to change their 'roles' in a cyclical manner under hormonal stimulation. In the mature human female, the ovaries are flat, bean-shaped organs measuring about 4 cm in length, 2 cm in width, and 1 cm in thickness. If examined in cross section, the ovary consists of two main compartments: an outer cortex and an inner medulla. The cortex, covered by a simple cuboidal epithelium, contains follicles at different stages of development. At any one time, some proportion of follicles in the mature female are developing, differentiating, or degenerating in a continuous process that lasts for the duration of a woman's reproductive life. Defects in tissue structure and function are associated with certain types of infertility, some of which are discussed here, and in more serious instances, with life-threatening cytopathologies that result in ovarian disease including cancer.

THE NORMAL HUMAN OVARY

Ovarian surface

A layer of mesothelial cells commonly referred to as the superficial epithelium covers the exposed surface of the ovary. This single continuous layer of polyhedral (columnar or flattened) cells is adorned with numerous microvilli, isolated cilia, and other specialized surface structures (Figure 38). This complex surface architecture undergoes dynamic change according to the phases of the reproductive cycle and levels of reproductive hormone activity[1,46–48]. Repair of cellular damage after ovulation requires that superficial cells in proximity to the ruptured follicle proliferate and migrate to the follicular apex to cover the rent created at the stigma where the oocyte and corresponding follicular contents were expelled. In the normal adult female, the density and distribution of the superficial epithelium can be highly variable and location-dependent and it does not form a complete covering. In the cycling human ovary, superficial cells appear to be concentrated in certain zones, mainly in the apical regions of the follicle prior to ovulation, and around the base and sides of the recently ovulated follicle. In contrast to the normally functioning ovary, the superficial epithelium in anovulatory women (see below) shows exceptional proliferative activity and exists as tightly packed cells that completely cover the ovary[10,47–50].

The surface of the ovary is not uniform but rather populated by numerous channel-like invaginations (clefts and crypts) and by truly remarkable projections, the papillae (Figures 39, 40). Clefts and papillae are highly variable in shape and size and arise from a common mechanism, the proliferation of the coelomic mesothelium. Some may be relatively transient formations whose spatial and temporal nature is an indication of the proliferative capability of the superficial epithelium under the influence of pituitary gonadotropins, ovarian steroids and other growth factors[10,48,50,51]. This notion is further supported by the occurrence of a vascular network within the papillae that can provide access to the circulatory system. These vessels may carry blood-borne growth factors that induce and support the growth of papillae and, if they remain patent, may provide a basis for some degree of permanence for these formations. While papillae are often covered by cells from the superficial epithelium, when viewed by SEM[48] these delicate structures can have a smooth acellular appearance (Figure 40) which may be indicative of their age, loss of vascularity, or their occurrence as residual structures that have yet to be resorbed.

Most epithelial ovarian carcinomas have been suggested to arise from the ovarian surface epithelium. The cyclical loss of integrity suffered by this epithelium at ovulation, in fact, might be followed by a stepwise or progressive sequence of genetic alterations. Even the formation of invaginations and inclusion cysts in the postovulatory period seems to be partly related to the pathogenesis of certain carcinomas. In particular, inclusion cysts are more frequently detected in ovaries contralateral to those containing malignant epithelial tumors than in normal ovaries[52].

Ovarian follicles

Follicles classified as 'resting' or in various phases of growth and development are embedded in the cortex of the ovary (Figure 41). As described in Chapter 1, a resting follicle consists of a small oocyte arrested in meiosis at the diplotene stage that is surrounded by a single layer of flattened follicular cells. Indeed, these so-called 'quiescent' oocytes can persist for decades in the human female, with some still detectable at the onset of menopause. Reticular nucleoli indicative of transcriptional capacity (RNA production) and extensive interactions between the oocyte and follicle cells are some of the unique submicroscopic features

of this stage of oogenesis that would appear to be inconsistent with the notion that resting or primordial follicular oocytes are truly quiescent (Figure 42).

Round or irregular mitochondria, Golgi vesicles and cisternae, membranes of endoplasmic reticulum, vacuoles, lipid droplets, compound aggregates (actually secondary lysosomes) and voluminous stacks of annulate lamellae are commonly found in the cytoplasm of the primordial oocytes. Most of these organelles occur in a characteristic crescent-shaped 'perinuclear complex' that has been traditionally termed Balbiani's vitelline body (Figure 42a, b)[53–55]. The occurrence of cytoplasmic stacks of nuclear membrane-like elements, the annulate lamellae, has been of particular interest to embryologists since they were first identified in oocytes decades ago. Annulate lamellae usually occur as parallel stacks of aligned (paired) membranes that result from multiple focal cytoplasmic replications of the nuclear envelope (Figure 42b). By TEM, they appear to have a higher porosity per unit of membrane than does the nuclear envelope and, in some sections, continuity between the annulate lamellae and outer leaflet of the nuclear membrane or the endoplasmic reticulum has been reported[53]. Kessel[55] suggests that the annulate lamellae may arise from blebbing of the outer leaflet of the nuclear membrane as it is periodically 'cast off' from the nucleus and subsequently aligns in the cytoplasm to simulate a nuclear envelope. Although the function of these assemblages is unclear, it has been suggested that the enormous amount of stacked and replicated nuclear membranes that occur with their pore complexes (or *annuli*) in perfect register may be a mechanism for transfer or storage of genetic information, perhaps in the form of an RNA[55]. The presence of annulate lamellae in oocytes arrested at the first meiotic prophase and in certain metabolically active somatic cells during interphase seems to be consistent with active nucleocytoplasmic trafficking processes[53,55,56]. Its occurrence in newly fertilized eggs may function in a manner similar to their counterparts in rapidly proliferating somatic cells (including tumor cells) where a specific 'reverse' transfer of membranes from the cytoplasm to the nucleus has been suggested. Evidence that the annulate lamellae promote normal pronuclear membrane formation in animal systems[57] is suggested for the human by fertilization arrest and early developmental failure when these elements are absent or have assembled in an apparently aberrant manner after *in vitro* fertilization[58].

The extraction of soluble cytoplasmic components is an important method in ultrastructural analysis because, when coupled with SEM, it can reveal fine details of the internal organization of cells. For human oocytes in resting and growing follicles, TEM provides an indication of the extent and type of interactions between follicular and germ cell compartments (Figure 43). For example, TEM demonstrates that the opposed surfaces of the oocyte and follicle cells are characterized by extensive interdigitation between microvilli elaborated by both cells (Figures 42c, 43), with specialized complexes, including gap junctions, clearly evident within these zones of intercellular contact (Figure 43b). TEM findings also suggest that elongated follicle cell projections may extend deeply into the human oocyte cytoplasm (Figures 42c, 43), often progressing as far as the nuclear membrane in some reconstructions of serial sections (Figure 42c)[1,11]. However, when imaged by SEM after cytoplasmic extraction (Figure 44), networks of microtubules can be seen coursing through the ooplasm where they appear to form a framework for intracellular organization in which mitochondria, elements of the endoplasmic reticulum and Golgi bodies are closely associated (Figures 45, 46). This method has been particularly useful in studying interactions between the oocyte and the surrounding somatic follicle cells (Figure 41), especially when older TEM studies provided basic insights into how these two compartments may communicate during the earliest stages of follicular growth. Cytoplasmic extraction and SEM analysis have confirmed this type of intercellular communication by enabling the tube-like follicle cell projections (FCP) to be identified in the ooplasm, where they are often observed in contact with mitochondria (Figure 45), Golgi complexes (Figure 46) and elements of the endoplasmic reticulum (Figure 47)[12]. While SEM images can provide a structural basis for the passage of proteins and other important low and high molecular weight molecules between oocyte and follicular compartments[1,11,12,21], the significance (or role) of this particular form of FCP-mediated intercellular communication in the regulation of oogenesis or folliculogenesis remains to be determined. The export of ATP to the oocyte is one possibility suggested by the association between fully developed mitochondria and networks of smooth endoplasmic reticulum (SER), especially those located in proximity to FCPs (Figure 48). Mitochondria–SER associations may be involved in the focal upregulation of respiration such that locally higher concentrations of ATP could be transferred to the oocyte through gap junctions between interdigitating microvilli or perhaps through those FCPs that appear to penetrate the ooplasm deeply[59].

Proximity of the primordial follicle to capillaries (Figure 42c) is of particular interest to those studying the regulation of oogenesis, as these vessels may serve as a mechanism to remove catabolites and a means by which blood-borne factors can be transmitted to follicle and germ cells. Although speculative, a link between maternal circulation, follicle cell and (by virtue of FCPs) the oocyte genome presents a physical conduit for information flow and signal transduction that may be of fundamental significance in the regulation of oogenesis and the determination of oocyte fate. It is well known that primordial follicles in the adult female undergo progressive depletion as the result of two processes: entry into the growth phase or, more commonly, atresia. How life or death pathways are determined for each follicle, and the extent to which, if any, this putative information flow pathway is involved in these decisions, are important questions that remain to be answered.

Follicular development

Cohorts of primordial follicles continuously enter the growth phase by regulatory processes that remain to be fully understood. In the human, it is estimated that over 100 days are required to complete development from the primordial to the fully grown (Graafian) preovulatory stage. As the oocyte grows and the number of surrounding layers of follicle cells increases, follicles progress through well-defined stages that allow them to be classified as primary, secondary (or antral) and tertiary (also termed preovulatory or Graafian)[54,60]. While the factors and mechanisms involved in follicular recruitment are poorly understood, development of the antral follicle to the preovulatory stage is well understood to be mediated by two pituitary protein hormones (gonadotropins), follicle stimulating hormone (FSH) and luteinizing hormone (LH).

The growth of the primary follicle is accompanied by a progressive thickening of the follicular wall and an increase in oocyte diameter[1,11,12,56]. For the oocyte, growth is accompanied by a corresponding increase in the density of cytoplasmic organelles, including a very significant expansion of the mitochondrial complement. However, for purposes of fertility treatment, the most relevant stage for detailed analysis occurs when the oocyte is fully grown and the follicle is competent to respond to FSH. It is to this cohort that current endocrine protocols are directed in order to promote the growth and maturation of multiple follicles and oocytes, respectively. For example, the goal of procedures used for clinical *in vitro* fertilization (IVF) is to obtain multiple mature oocytes that are capable of developing into competent embryos in culture and which retain competence after transfer to the uterus. Consequently, it is the development of the follicles under the influence of FSH and LH that is of primary importance in clinical treatments of infertility and as such is emphasized here.

The development of the antral follicle

Normal follicular growth requires the simultaneous enlargement of the oocyte and an increase in the number of associated follicular cells. As the follicle grows, follicular cells (termed granulosa cells) proliferate and become stratified in an increasing number of layers to form the so-called stratum granulosum. This granulosa layer is one of the most dynamic epithelia in the human female body because its characteristics and functions in preantral and antral follicles are transient and specifically influenced by changing hormonal conditions and levels[51,61]. The granulosa layer has an essential role in the formation of follicular fluid[62], whose increase in volume causes the expansion of the oocyte-containing cyst known as the follicular antrum (Figures 49, 50a). Subpopulations of these cells synthesize a variety of potent growth factors, steroid hormones and other regulatory molecules that accumulate in the follicular fluid and have important influences on the progression and normality of oocyte and follicle development and function[63]. The fluid also contains transudates from perifollicular capillaries that, in combination with endogenously synthesized bioactive molecules and growth factors, form a biochemically complex intrafollicular environment that changes quantitatively and qualitatively under the influence of FSH and LH. Differences in composition between follicles in the same ovary have been related to differential effects on oocyte competence[64].

Under the influence of FSH, the antrum increases in size, and the oocyte with its surrounding layer of granulosa cells (so-called oocyte–cumulus complex) is usually displaced to one portion of the follicular wall (Figures 49, 50). During the FSH-dominated follicular phase of the menstrual cycle, the granulosa cells are compartmentalized into two basic regions: the mural granulosa that lines the wall of the follicle and the cumulus granulosa that surrounds the oocyte. These compartments have distinct and different biosynthetic activities, with estrogen produced primarily by the mural granulosa and certain potent regulatory growth factors produced by the cumulus granulosa (cumulus oophorus, Figure 50)[63]. The complete development of the follicle is associated with an increase in granulosa cell numbers from approximately 1000 to nearly 1 000 000.

The nature of the communication between oocyte and cumulus granulosa is one of the more important questions in current studies of mammalian oogenesis, as it is now clear that protein growth factors synthesized by and released from the oocyte regulate follicular development and vice versa[59,65]. In the human, an understanding of how this communication may be involved in the establishment of developmental competence after fertilization has become a critical issue in infertility treatments that involve controlled ovarian hyperstimulation and IVF. In the preantral and antral follicle, the extent of contact between the cumulus mass of follicular cells and the oocyte is limited by the zona pellucida, a protein shell-like layer that develops during earlier stages of oogenesis[1,9,11,18,21,54,60,61]. Unlike the very extensive interdigitation of opposing microvilli described above for primary follicles, direct communication between somatic and germ cell compartments in secondary and more advanced follicles is largely maintained by means of numerous elongated projections known as follicle cell (FCP) or transzonal processes (TZP). These cellular projections extend through the zona pellucida from a layer of cumulus granulosa cells (termed the corona radiata) that generally resides on the zona surface, and are thought to be 'fixed' in a permanent position when the zona pellucida forms from proteins secreted by the growing oocyte. These elongated and branching processes contact the oocyte plasma membrane and maintain bidirectional intercellular communication and molecular transport by means of endocytotic/exocytotic mechanisms and, more importantly, cell surface specializations such as gap junctions[59]. In addition to active bidirectional molecular trafficking between cumulus/corona cells and the oocyte, TZPs are also involved in the regulation of the meiotic resumption during the preovulatory phase of oogenesis[1,11,12,66]. If the oocyte and zona pellucida are dissolved *in situ*, SEM imaging of the residual FCPs/TZPs originating from the corona radiata (asterisk, Figure 51) provides a clear indication of the extensive network of slender cellular projections that the oocyte actually 'sees' *in vivo*, especially at higher magnifications (Figure 52). The extent and complexity of this cellular network can be fully appreciated by SEM methods such as those used to produce Figures 51 and 52. It is images of this type that clearly demonstrate the structural basis for potentially robust interactions and molecular exchange between the oocyte and a subset of follicle cells that surround the zona pellucida.

THE PREOVULATORY HUMAN FOLLICLE

The release of LH from the pituitary marks the end of the follicular phase and beginning of the luteal phase of the menstrual cycle. This release occurs rapidly and, because an abrupt elevation of LH can be detected in the circulatory system, it has long been known as 'the LH surge'. In the human female, ovulation occurs approximately 36–40 hours after the LH surge reaches its maximum level. In cycles of infertility treatment that use controlled ovarian stimulation, multiple follicles are induced to ovulate by the administration of human chorionic gonadotropin (hCG) but, for IVF procedures, the oocyte and the corresponding pool of follicular fluid are withdrawn (termed follicular aspiration) through a needle under ultrasound guidance. Much of what we currently understand about the morphology and morphodynamics of the preovulatory follicle comes from clinical procedures including those in which follicular growth and ovulation were timed by exogenous management of the menstrual cycle. In this respect, SEM is an ideal method to detect differences in cell surface architecture that may be related to differential cell function during the menstrual cycle or to pathologies that may be associated with infertility.

Alterations in the surface architecture of granulosa cells are one of the most evident of cellular changes detectable by SEM in preovulatory human follicles. These changes occur in response to hormonal stimulation and are thought to reflect an expansion of cell surface area associated with enhanced gonadotropin binding[67–69]. Figure 53a is a low magnification SEM image of a preovulatory human Graafian follicle that has been manipulated to reveal internal details. The layer of steroid hormone producing mural granulosa occurs in a series of folds and, at higher magnification, the oval shape of these cells is apparent, as are tufts of elongated microvilli elaborated from their apical surface (Figure 53b). In contrast, cells of the cumulus oophorus that enclose the oocyte are largely spherical (Figure 53c). The basal layer of the mural granulosa cells appears to be firmly adhered to the follicular wall by cellular extensions that interact with collagen fibers embedded in the basement membrane (Figure 54a)[61]. The secretory nature of the mural granulosa cells is suggested by a surface architecture containing pseudopodium-like processes and numerous surface expansions (Figure 54b). For these cells, a higher density of LH receptors and a shift in steroid production from estrogen to progesterone are accompanied by an increased number of secretory bleb-like structures and long, slender microvilli (Figure 55a)[47,70]. By TEM (Figure 55b), the cytoplasm of mural granulosa cells in preovulatory follicles contains arrays of rough-surfaced endoplasmic reticulum, mitochondria with tubular cristae and electron-dense inclusions representing lipid and/or luteal bodies. These subcellular characteristics are typical of steroid-secreting granulosa cells in general and those undergoing the transition from estrogen to progesterone secretion in particular[51,61,71,72].

As imaged by SEM, the surface or superficial epithelium at the apex of normal human preovulation is populated by numerous exfoliating cells that are interconnected by thin cytoplasmic extensions and organized so that large areas of the basement membrane are exposed (Figure 56). As shown in this figure, these exfoliating cells have a unique 'mulberry' appearance that has been suggested to reflect a dense accumulation of spherical lysosomes within the cortical cytoplasm[47,48,61]. Alternatively, this appearance may represent a premorbid or moribund state associated with degenerative or apoptotic processes. Indeed, the decomposition of the intercellular ground substance at the follicular apex may be the result of the normal secretion of lytic enzymes by intact cells or their release as a consequence of cellular deterioration. The focal elimination of the superficial epithelium, the exposure of the underlying basement membrane and tunica albuginea (TA, Figure 56), the dissociation of collagen fibers and proteins, and degradation of perifollicular capillaries in proximity to the follicular apex, are destructive processes that are a normal aspect of the preovulatory stage and necessary prerequisites for ovulation[2,73].

The postovulatory follicle and formation of the corpus luteum

In specimens fixed for SEM, a veil of dense precipitated material consisting of follicular and interstitial fluids and cellular debris often obscures the oocyte, which is enclosed by the cumulus oophorus (commonly termed the oocyte–cumulus complex or OCC). Because ovulation can occur rather abruptly (within minutes), it is rare for SEM analysis of this process to be so precisely timed as to obtain views of the OCC during its expulsion from the follicle. Indeed, published images of the ovulatory process obtained from animal models such as the rabbit and mouse used superovulation techniques and numerous ovaries that were systematically fixed at closely timed intervals after ovulation induction to obtain such images[2,73]. While similar studies cannot be undertaken for the human, it is likely that the underlying processes detectable by SEM in animal models also apply to women. For example, findings from both animal models and women show that the superficial cells surrounding the stigma – the site at the apex where follicular rupture occurs – become flattened, irregular in shape and size and, as ovulation approaches, slough off in discrete monolayers. After ovulation, ragged layers of residual superficial epithelium project into the rent created during ovulation, demonstrating that the expulsion of the oocyte can be associated with considerable cellular damage and tissue disruption at the follicular stigma (Figure 57a). Changes in geometry and surface architecture in regions of undamaged superficial epithelium in proximity to the stigma that are associated with follicular repair are consistent with rapid cell division and migration to disrupted regions. In regions slightly more distant from their migratory counterparts, the occurrence of large numbers of cells interconnected by numerous slender filopodia indicates zones of active mitotic proliferation (Figure 57b). Intermixed within domains of actively dividing cells are cells whose ruffled plasma membrane morphology (Figure 58) may be related to active secretion and/or endocytosis[10,46–48,51,61,74]. Repair of the rent created at

ovulation is an essential first step in the postovulatory phase. The diverse cellular phenotypes detected in the disrupted regions of the relatively few postovulatory human ovaries that have been examined by SEM are similar to images obtained from animal models and indicative of intense mitotic and biosynthetic activities common in wound healing.

For the follicle, ovulation is followed by the transformation of the residual mural granulosa cells into progesterone-secreting luteal cells. Strands of connective tissue containing capillaries form a delicate network around groups of luteal cells, creating a dense core of connective tissue and a direct mechanism for progesterone transport into the circulatory system. Indeed, one of the most important prerequisites for an ongoing pregnancy is the detection of rising levels of serum progesterone that originate from the transformed luteal cells. This is especially important in clinical IVF where the precise time of conception is known and, after embryo transfer, rising progesterone levels signal the embryonic production of hCG which upregulates progesterone production by luteal cells and mediates the transformation of these cells into a functional endocrine organ, the corpus luteum. The typical luteal cell cytoplasm is densely packed with lipid droplets, polymorphic lysosomes and autophagic vacuoles (Figure 59a, b). As these cells proliferate, the resulting corpus luteum appears as a solid body of glandular cells[1,61,71] that, when viewed in cross section by SEM, has a honeycomb appearance in which luteal cells are surrounded by a dense connective tissue (Figure 59c). The lifespan of a corpus luteum is determined by whether or not pregnancy is established. If a viable embryo implants and progresses through gestation, the corpus luteum enlarges and actively secretes progesterone for several months. If fertilization or implantation has not occurred, or embryo demise is accompanied by the cessation of hCG synthesis and secretion, the corpus luteum persists for several days and then regresses as the luteal cells degenerate, their endocrine activity ceases, and the current menstrual cycle terminates[1,9,74,75].

Ovarian pathology related to infertility

Polycystic ovarian disease (PCOD) and luteinized unruptured follicle (LUF) syndrome are two conditions associated with anovulatory cycles and infertility in women. PCOD is characterized by menstrual abnormalities and clinical or biochemical features of hyperandrogenism, which include obesity, hirsutism, glucose intolerance, hyperlipidemia and cardiovascular disease. PCOD is caused by a variety of dysfunctions of which disorders of the hypothalamic–pituitary–ovarian axis are the most common, although adrenal androgens or ovarian androgen-producing tumors can be involved. PCOD is the consequence of a relatively constant LH stimulation that enlarges the ovaries and produces a polycystic condition owing to the presence of numerous growing follicles that are incapable of ovulation. The granulosa layer is greatly affected by this condition so that the production of estrogens is significantly reduced. Conversely, cells comprising the theca interna may become hyperplastic with hormonal synthesis shifted towards androgen production. LUF is another anovulatory condition in which follicular luteinizing and progesterone production occur in the absence of ovulation and oocyte release. While anovulatory cycles do occur periodically in normally fertile women, persistent or chronic episodes of LUF are more frequent in infertile women with endometriosis and pelvic inflammation.

The ovarian surface

The surface epithelium of the normal human ovary is often discontinuous and normally shows differences in cell density and organization, such as in the apical regions of the preovulatory follicle. With the exception of regions associated with postovulatory follicles, the superficial epithelium does not exhibit significant proliferative activity. In contrast, a highly proliferative and tightly packed superficial epithelium that completely covers the ovary is one of the most characteristic features of anovulatory women that has been revealed by SEM. Superficial cells showing signs of growth and proliferation that include blebs, ruffles and filopodia (Figure 60) are particularly evident in women with PCOD[10,47–50,61] and probably reflect constitutively elevated levels of LH. This abnormally high proliferative capacity is especially evident at the apex of abnormal cystic follicles in PCOD patients (Figure 61). It has been proposed that the widespread occurrence of ruffles (also known as lamellipodia) on the surface epithelium of polycystic ovaries may reflect pathological levels of endocytosis, a normal process by which substances are incorporated into the cells without passing

through the usual mechanisms of cell membrane-mediated uptake (Figure 62)[47,61]. As a consequence of the enhanced proliferative activity of the superficial epithelium under abnormal hormonal conditions, papillae in PCOD patients are larger and more numerous (Figure 63) than in normal women[47,48,61]. SEM analysis of ovaries from LUF syndrome patients shows a superficial epithelium that is densely adorned by microvilli and contains numerous clusters of smooth-surfaced cells in the S phase of mitosis (Figure 64). As noted above, these are features of a highly proliferative cell layer that are not observed in normal human ovaries[46,47,61].

Anovulatory follicles

Anovulatory follicles also show an abnormal internal architecture by SEM. In follicles of PCOD patients, the mural granulosa layer rapidly degenerates leaving patches of granulosa cells in scattered clusters unevenly distributed along the basement membrane of the follicle (asterisk, Figure 65a). The granulosa layer may be disrupted, with blood cells and macrophages invading the antrum. In these cases, the theca interna is usually formed by hypertrophic cells supplied by an extensive capillary network, whereas the theca externa shows widespread collagenous fibers and fibroblast formation[47,51,76]. In advanced stages of PCOD, granulosa cells become smooth-surfaced, irregular in size and shape and exhibit occasional distorted microvilli blebs (Figure 65b). However, some cells are seen with long, slender microvilli and blebs of various sizes (Figure 65c). The detection of these surface features suggests that some residual granulosa cells in follicles from advanced stage PCOD can still undergo luteinization and produce progesterone[47,51,76].

REFERENCES – SECTION ONE

1. Motta PM, Nottola SA, Familiari G, Makabe S, Stallone T, Macchiarelli G. Morphodynamics of the follicular–luteal complex during early ovarian development and reproductive life. Int Rev Cytol 2003; 223: 177–288

2. Van Blerkom J, Motta PM. The Cellular Basis of Mammalian Reproduction. Baltimore: Urban & Schwarzenberg, 1979

3. Van Blerkom J, Motta PM. Ultrastructure of Human Gametogenesis and Early Embryogenesis. Boston: Kluwer Academic Publishers, 1989

4. Motta PM. Developments in Ultrastructure of Reproduction. New York: Alan R Liss, 1989. Prog Clin Biol Res 296

5. Motta PM. Microscopy of Reproduction and Development: A Dynamic Approach. Rome: A Delfino Editore, 1997

6. Familiari G, Makabe S, Motta PM. Ultrastructure of the Ovary. Boston: Kluwer Academic Publishers, 1991

7. Macchiarelli G, Nottola SA, Correr S, Motta PM. New Trends in Microanatomy of Reproduction. Marcello Malpighi Symposia Series, Vol VI. Florence: Il Sedicesimo, 1998. Ital J Anat Embryol 103 (Suppl 1)

8. Motta PM, Nottola SA, Macchiarelli G, Correr S. Molecular, Cellular and Developmental Biology of Reproduction. Basic and Clinical Aspects. Marcello Malpighi Symposia Series, Vol VIII. Florence: Il Sedicesimo, 2001. Ital J Anat Embryol 106 (Suppl 2)

9. Motta PM, Makabe S. An Atlas of Menopausal Aging. Lancaster: Parthenon Publishing, 2003

10. Motta PM, Van Blerkom J, Makabe S. Changes in the surface morphology of ovarian 'germinal' epithelium during the reproductive cycle and in some pathological conditions. J Submicrosc Cytol 1980; 12: 407–25

11. Motta PM, Makabe S, Naguro T, Correr S. Oocyte follicle cells association during development of human ovarian follicle. A study by high resolution scanning and transmission electron microscopy. Arch Histol Cytol 1994; 57: 369–94

12. Makabe S, Naguro T, Motta PM. A new approach to the study of ovarian follicles by scanning electron microscopy and ODO maceration. Arch Histol Cytol 1992; 55 (Suppl): 183–90

13. Motta PM, Makabe S. Development of the ovarian surface and associated germ cells in the human fetus. A correlated study by scanning and transmission electron microscopy. Cell Tissue Res 1982; 226: 493–510

14. Motta PM, Makabe S. Elimination of germ cells during differentiation of the human ovary: an electron microscopic study. Eur J Obstet Gynecol 1986; 22: 271–86

15. Motta PM, Makabe S. Germ cells in the ovarian surface during fetal development in humans. A three-dimensional microanatomical study by scanning and transmission electron microscopy. J Submicrosc Cytol 1986; 18: 271–90

16. Makabe S, Motta PM. Migration of human germ cells and their relationship with the developing ovary: ultrastructural aspects. Prog Clin Biol Res 1989; 296: 41–54

17. Makabe S, Nottola SA, Motta PM. Life history of the human female germ cell: ultrastructural aspects. In

Van Blerkom J, Motta PM, eds. Ultrastructure of Human Gametogenesis and Early Embryogenesis. Boston: Kluwer Academic Publishers, 1989: 33–60

18. Makabe S, Naguro T, Nottola SA, Pereda J, Motta PM. Migration of germ cells, development of the ovary, and folliculogenesis. In Familiari G, Makabe S, Motta PM, eds. Ultrastructure of the Ovary. Boston: Kluwer Academic Publishers, 1991: 1–27

19. Motta PM, Makabe S, Nottola SA. The ultrastructure of human reproduction. I. The natural history of the female germ cell: origin, migration and differentiation inside the developing ovary. Hum Reprod Update 1997; 3: 281–95

20. Motta PM, Nottola SA, Makabe S. Natural history of the female germ cell from its origin to full maturation through prenatal ovarian development. Eur J Obstet Gynecol 1997; 75: 5–10

21. Motta PM, Nottola SA, Makabe S, Heyn R. Mitochondrial morphology in human fetal and adult female germ cells. Hum Reprod 2000; 15 (Suppl 2): 129–47

22. Nottola SA, Makabe S, Stallone T, et al. Ultrastructure and distribution of interstitial cells in human fetal ovaries. Arch Histol Cytol 2000; 63: 345–55

23. Tanaka K, Naguro T. High resolution scanning electron microscopy of cell organelles by a new specimen preparation method. Biomed Res 1981; 2: 63–70

24. McLaren A. Germ and somatic cell lineages in the developing gonad. Mol Cell Endocrinol 2000; 163: 3–9

25. Viebahn C, Miething A, Wartenberg H. Primordial germ cells of the rabbit are specifically recognized by a monoclonal antibody labelling the perimitochondrial cytoplasm. Histochem Cell Biol 1998; 109: 49–58

26. Edwards RG. New approaches to achieving human fertilization: a resume. Hum Reprod 1998; 13: 127–36, discussion 145–7

27. Donovan PJ. Primordial germ cells. In Knobil E, Neill JD, eds. Encyclopedia of Reproduction, Vol III. London: Academic Press, 1999: 1064–72

28. Anderson R, Fassler R, Georges-Labouesse E, et al. Mouse primordial germ cells lacking beta1 integrins enter the germline but fail to migrate normally to the gonads. Development 1999; 126: 1655–64

29. De Felici M. Regulation of primordial germ cell development in the mouse. Int J Dev Biol 2000; 44 (6 Spec No): 575–80

30. Kierszenbaum AL, Tres LL. Primordial germ cell–somatic cell partnership: a balancing cell signaling act. Mol Reprod Dev 2001; 60: 277–80

31. Soto-Suazo M, Abrahamsohn PA, Pereda J, et al. Modulation of hyaluronan in the migratory pathway

of mouse primordial germ cells. Histochem Cell Biol 2002; 117: 265–73

32. Wakayama T, Hamada K, Yamamoto M, Suda T, Iseki S. The expression of platelet endothelial cell adhesion molecule-1 in mouse primordial germ cells during their migration and early gonadal formation. Histochem Cell Biol 2003; 119: 355–62

33. Stallock J, Molyneaux K, Schaible K, Knudson CM, Wylie C. The pro-apoptotic gene bax is required for the death of ectopic primordial germ cells during their migration in the mouse embryo. Development 2003; 130: 6589–97

34. Donovan PJ, de Miguel MP. Turning germ cells into stem cells. Curr Opin Genet Dev 2003; 13: 463–71

35. Sathananthan AH, Selvaraj K, Trounson A. Fine structure of human oogonia in the foetal ovary. Mol Cell Endocrinol 2000; 161: 3–8

36. Van Blerkom J, Motta PM. Fertilization and preimplantation embryogenesis. In Van Blerkom J, Motta PM, eds. The Cellular Basis of Mammalian Reproduction. Baltimore: Urban & Schwarzenberg, 1979: 165–89

37. Eddy EM. The germ line and development. Dev Genet 1996; 19: 287–9

38. Motta P, Van Blerkom J. Presence d'un materiel caracteristique granulaire dans le cytoplasma de l'ovocyte et dans les premiers stades de la differenciation des cellules embryonnaires. Bull Assoc Anat (Nancy) 1974; 58: 350–5

39. Pepling ME, Spradling AC. Mouse ovarian germ cell cysts undergo programmed breakdown to form primordial follicles. Dev Biol 2001; 234: 339–51

40. Hoang-Ngoc Minh, Makabe S, Nottola SA, Smadja A, Motta PM. La folliculogenese au cours de l'organogenese ovarienne humaine. Gynecologie 1993; 44: 67–80

41. Sawyer HR, Smith P, Heath DA, Juengel JL, Wakefield SJ, McNatty KP. Formation of ovarian follicles during fetal development in sheep. Biol Reprod 2002; 66: 1134–50

42. Tilly JL. The molecular basis of ovarian cell death during germ cell attrition, follicular atresia, and luteolysis. Front Biosci 1996; 1: d1–11

43. De Pol A, Vaccina F, Forabosco A, Cavazzuti E, Marzona L. Apoptosis of germ cells during human prenatal oogenesis. Hum Reprod 1997; 12: 2235–41

44. Johnson J, Canning J, Kaneko K, Pru JK, Tilly JL. Germline stem cells and follicular renewal in the postnatal mammalian ovary. Nature 2004; 428: 145–50

45. Bukovsky A, Caudle MR, Svetlikova M, Upadhyaya NB. Origin of germ cells and formation of new primary follicles in adult human ovaries. Reprod Biol Endocrinol 2004; 2: 20

46. Porter KR, Prescott D, Frye J. Changes in the surface morphology of Chinese hamster ovary cells during the cell cycle. J Cell Biol 1973; 57: 815–36

47. Makabe S. Scanning electron microscopy of normal and anovulatory human ovaries. Eleventh International Congress of Anatomy. In Vidrio EA, Galina MA, eds. Advances in the Morphology of Cells and Tissues. New York: Alan R Liss, 1981: 321–30

48. Makabe S. Scanning electron microscopy of normal and anovulatory human ovaries. In Allen DJ, Motta PM, DiDio LJA, eds. Three Dimensional Microanatomy of Cells and Tissue Surfaces. Amsterdam: Elsevier, 1981: 245–66

49. Makabe S, Shibata N, Iwaki A, Hafez ESE, Motta P. Human ovaries as viewed by scanning electron microscopy. Proceedings IXth World Congress of Gynecology–Obstetrics, Tokyo, 1979: 101–2

50. Makabe S, Iwaki A, Hafez ESE, Motta P. Physiomorphology of human ovaries. In Motta PM, Hafez ESE, eds. Biology of the Ovary. The Hague: Martinus Nijhoff, 1980: 279–90

51. Motta PM, Makabe S. Morphodynamic changes of the mammalian ovary in normal and some pathological conditions. Biomed Res 1981; 2 (Suppl): 325–39

52. Katabuchi H, Okamura H. Cell biology of human ovarian surface epithelial cells and ovarian carcinogenesis. Med Electron Microsc 2003; 36: 74–86

53. Hertig AT. Some observations on the fine structure of Balbiani's vitelline body and the origin of the annulate lamellae. Am J Anat 1968; 122: 107–37

54. Dvorak M, Tesarik J. Ultrastructure of human ovarian follicles. In Motta PM, Hafez ESE, eds. Biology of the Ovary. The Hague: Martinus Nijhoff, 1980: 121–37

55. Kessel RG. Annulate lamellae: a last frontier in cellular organelles. Int Rev Cytol 1992; 133: 43–120

56. Baca M, Zamboni L. The fine structure of human follicular oocytes. J Ultrastruct Res 1967; 19: 354–81

57. Sutovsky P, Simerly C, Hewitson L, Schatten G. Assembly of nuclear pore complexes and annulate lamellae promotes normal pronuclear development in fertilized mammalian oocytes. J Cell Sci 1998; 111: 2841–54

58. Rawe VY, Olmedo SB, Nodar FN, Ponzio R, Sutovsky P. Abnormal assembly of annulate lamellae and nuclear pore complexes coincides with fertilization arrest at the pronuclear stage of human zygotic development. Hum Reprod 2003; 18: 576–82

59. Albertini D. Oocyte–granulosa cell interactions. In Van Blerkom J, Gregory L, eds. Essential IVF: Basic Research and Clinical Applications. Norwell, MA: Kluwer Academic Publishers, 2004: 43–58

60. Franchi LL, Baker TG. Oogenesis and follicular growth. In Hafez ESE, Evans TN, eds. Human Reproduction. New York: Harper and Row, 1973: 53–83

61. Familiari G, Makabe S, Motta PM. The ovary and ovulation: a three-dimensional ultrastructural study. In Van Blerkom J, Motta PM, eds. Ultrastructure of Human Gametogenesis and Early Embryogenesis. Boston: Kluwer Academic Publishers, 1989: 85–124

62. Motta P, Van Blerkom J. Structure and ultrastructure of ovarian follicles. In Hafez ESE, ed. Human Ovulation. North-Holland, Amsterdam: Elsevier, 1979: 17–38

63. Antczak M. The synthetic and secretory behaviors (nonsteroidal) of ovarian follicular granulosa cells: parallels to cells of the endothelial cell lineage. In Van Blerkom J, Gregory L, eds. Essential IVF: Basic Research and Clinical Applications. Norwell, MA: Kluwer Academic Publishers, 2004: 1–41

64. Michael A. Do biochemical predictors of IVF outcome exist? In Van Blerkom J, Gregory L, eds. Essential IVF: Basic Research and Clinical Applications. Norwell, MA: Kluwer Academic Publishers, 2004: 81–109

65. Eppig J. Oocyte control of ovarian follicular development and function in mammals. Reproduction 2001; 122: 829–38

66. Makabe S, Naguro T, Motta PM. Ovarian follicles studied by scanning electron microscopy and osmium–dimethylsulfoxide–osmium maceration method. In Sjoberg NO, Hamberger L, Janson PO, Owman Ch, Coelingh Bennink HJT, eds. Local Regulation of Ovarian Function. Carnforth, UK: Parthenon Publishing, 1991: 117–21

67. Amsterdam A, Koch Y, Liebermann E, Linder HR. Distribution of binding sites for human chorionic gonadotropin in the preovulatory follicle of the rat. J Cell Biol 1975; 67: 894–9

68. Makabe S, Hafez ESE. Scanning electron microscopy of ovulation. In: Hafez ESE, ed. Human Ovulation. Amsterdam: Elsevier, North-Holland 1979: 39–53

69. Motta PM. Ovulation: a three-dimensional correlative analysis by scanning and transmission electron microscopy. In Zichella L, Pancheri P, eds. Psychoneuroendocrinology in Reproduction, Vol V. Amsterdam: Elsevier, North-Holland 1979: 145–55

70. Ryan RJ, Lee CY. The role of membrane bound receptors. Biol Reprod 1976; 14: 16–29

71. Makabe S, Hafez ESE, Motta P. The ovary and ovulation. In Hafez ESE, Kenemans P, eds. Atlas of Human Reproduction by Scanning Electron Microscopy. Lancaster: MTP Press, 1982: 135–44

72. Makabe S, Kaneko Y, Kojima E, Omura G, Momose K. The human granulosa cell changes during luteogenesis viewed by scanning and transmission electron microscopy. In Harrison RF, Bonnar J, Thompson W, eds. In Vitro Fertilization, Embryo Transfer and Early Pregnancy. Lancaster: MTP Press, 1983: 33–6

73. Motta PM, Van Blerkom J. A scanning electron microscopic study of the luteo-follicular complex. II. Events leading to ovulation. Am J Anat 1975; 143: 241–63

74. Van Blerkom J, Motta PM. A scanning electron microscopic study of the luteo-follicular complex. III. Formation of the corpus luteum and repair of the ovulated follicle. Cell Tissue Res 1978; 189: 131–54

75. Motta P, Andrews PM, Porter KR. Microanatomy of Cells and Tissue Surfaces. An Atlas of Scanning Electron Microscopy. Philadelphia: Lea & Febiger, 1977: 144–63

76. Peluso JJ, Steger RW, Hafez ESE. Surface ultrastructural changes in granulosa cells of atretic follicles. Biol Reprod 1977; 16: 600–4

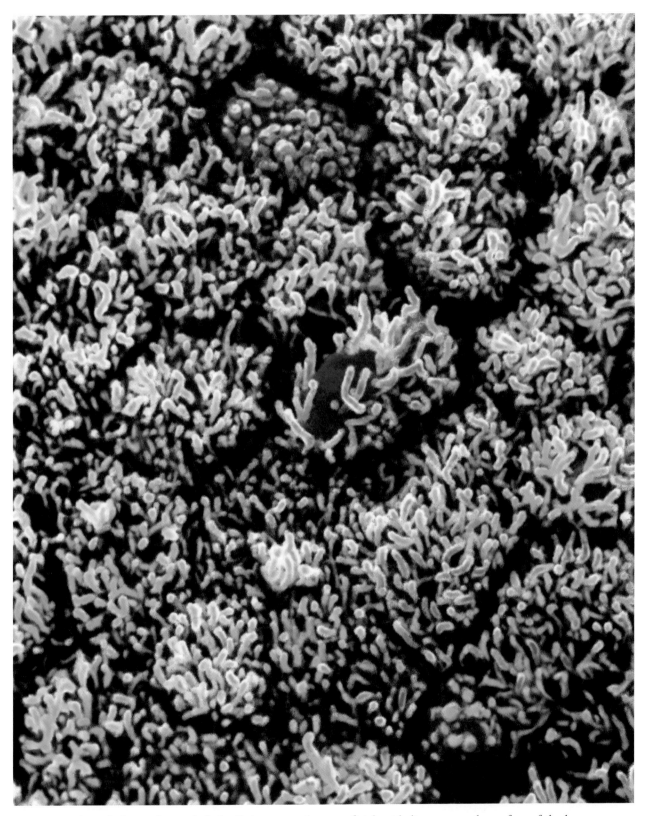

Figure 38 A single layer of mesothelial cells known as the superficial epithelium covers the surface of the human ovary. It is a functionally complex and dynamic epithelium that responds to cyclic hormonal and environmental changes during the menstrual cycle and is involved in ovulation and repair of tissue damage at the follicular apex after ovulation. A dense complement of microvilli and scattered cilia are the characteristic surface features of this epithelium as revealed by SEM

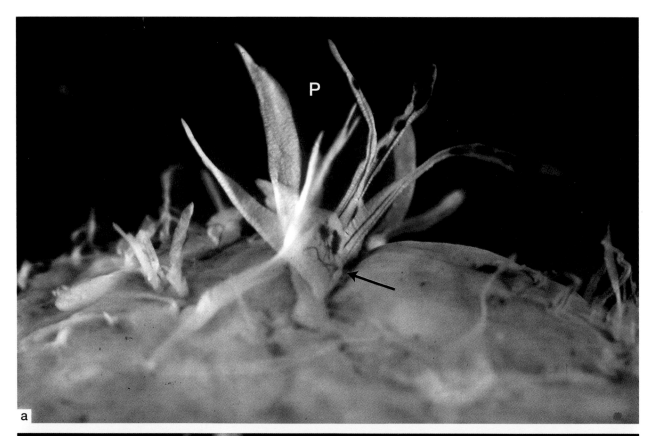

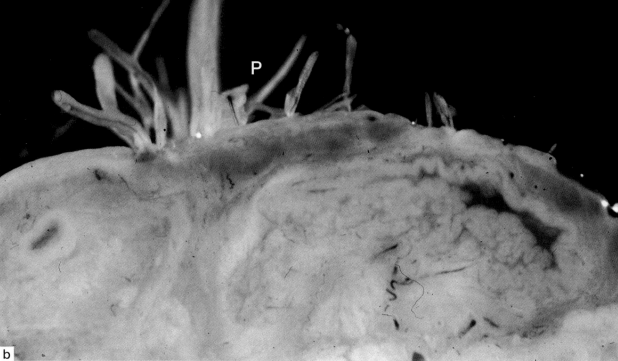

Figure 39 Papillae are one of the more remarkable features detected on the surface of the human ovary. These villus-like structures (P) arise from the ovarian surface as vascularized (arrow, a) projections from the underlying cortex. Differences in density and size are considered indicators of the proliferative capability of the superficial epithelium under the influence of pituitary gonadotropins and ovarian steroids. (b) shows a follicle in which a corpus luteum has developed after ovulation. The proliferative activity of the superficial epithelium that is involved in follicular repair is evident by the expression of numerous papillae at the apex of this follicle

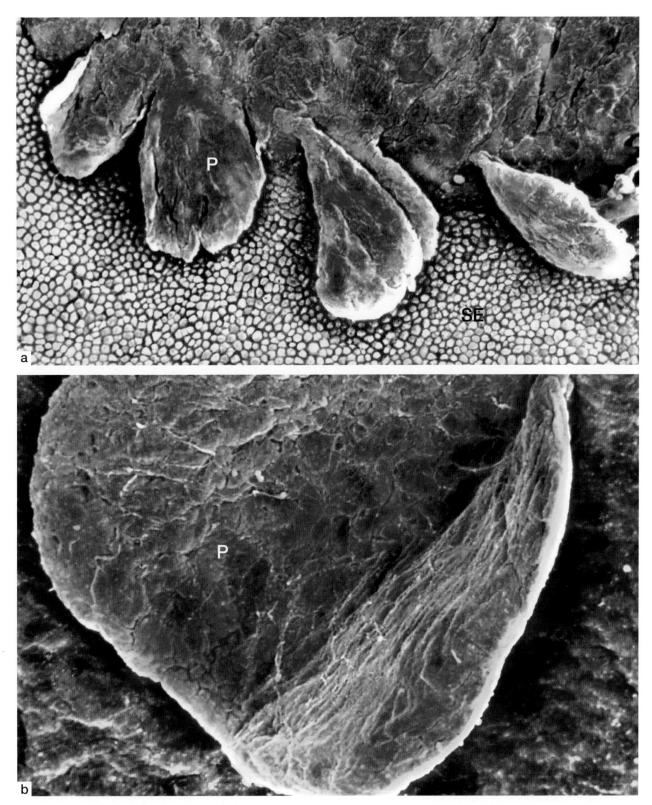

Figure 40 (a) is an SEM image of branching papillae (P) at the apex of a newly formed corpus luteum in which the superficial epithelium (SE) appears absent while such cells are clearly evident as a cobblestone-like layer immediately beneath the papillae. The apparent absence of a superficial epithelium is shown at higher magnification in (b)

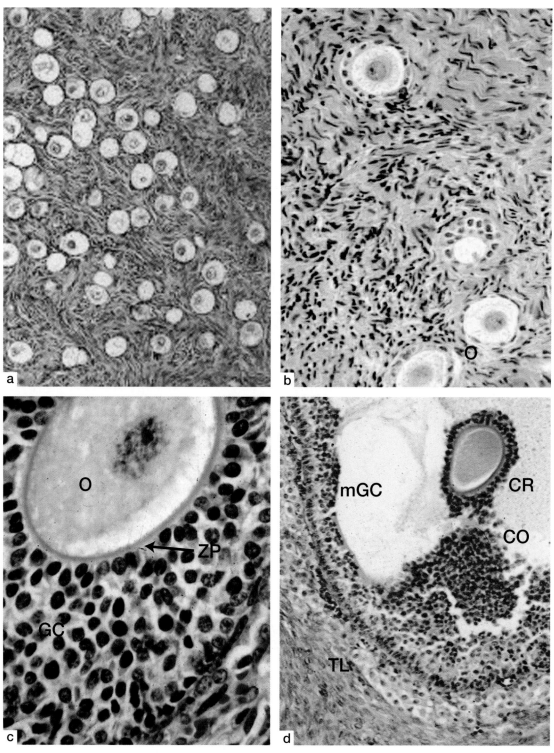

Figure 41   A series of light micrographs of follicles at different stages of development. For comparative purposes, (a) shows the high-density distribution of oogonia and oocytes in an 18-week-old human ovary while, in the adult ovary, the density of germ cells (primordial oocytes) is significantly reduced (b). (c) shows a growing oocyte (O) surrounded by multiple layers of granulosa cells (GC) in a late secondary follicle. A distinct zona pellucida (ZP, arrow) is observable at the interface between oocyte and granulosa cells. The growth of the preovulatory Graafian follicle is characterized by the accumulation of fluid and the formation of the antrum (d). During the progressive expansion of the follicle, the steroid-producing mural granulosa cells that line the follicular wall (mGC) can be clearly distinguished from the granulosa cells associated with the oocyte, which occur as two elements: the corona radiata (CR) which directly surrounds the oocyte; and the more distal cells of the cumulus oophorus (CO). A concentric arrangement of the stromal cells that form the thecal layers (TL) just outside the mural granulosa compartment is also evident

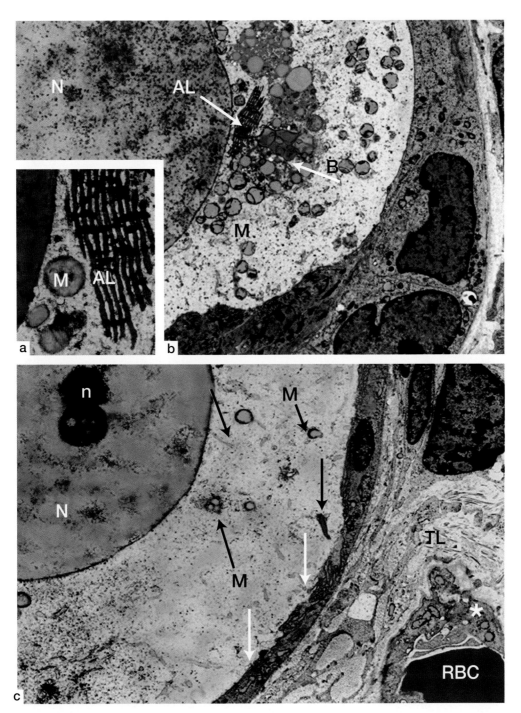

Figure 42 In the adult ovary, primordial follicles occur through the cortex although their numbers decrease significantly with advanced reproductive age. (a) Oocytes in primordial follicles observed in the adult ovary contain a characteristic aggregation of perinuclear organelles known as Balbiani's vitelline body (B) that is composed of mitochondria (M), lipid droplets, lysosomes, endoplasmic reticulum membranes and stacks of annulate lamellae (AL, b). The voluminous stacks of annulate lamellae are derived from the nuclear membrane and are considered an ultrastructural indication of active nucleo-cytoplasmic transfer. Prior to the formation of the zona pellucida during the earliest stages of oogenesis, the oocyte in an 'intermediary' follicle, i.e. between primordial and primary stages, is surrounded by a monolayer of somatic follicle cells. Intercellular communication between germ and somatic cells involves extensive interconnected microvilli (white arrows, c) and longer cellular projections elaborated by both cell types. Indeed, serial thin section analysis demonstrates that cytoplasmic projections from follicle cells deeply penetrate the oocyte cytoplasm (c), with some traceable from the oocyte plasma membrane (black arrows) to the oocyte nuclear membrane. An evident nucleolus (n) is seen in the oocyte nucleus (N). Scattered mitochondria (M) are found in the oocyte cytoplasm. An arteriole (asterisk) containing a red blood cell (RBC) is seen in the developing thecal layer (TL)

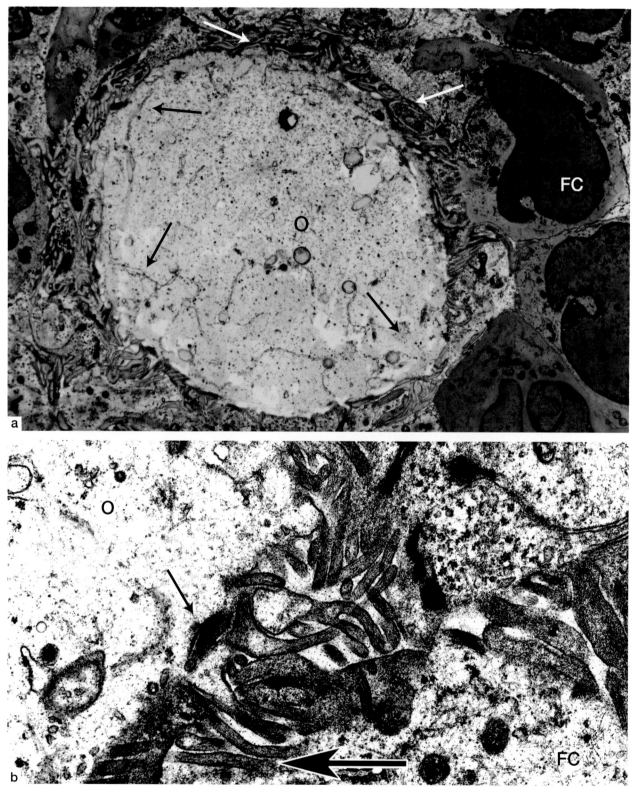

Figure 43   These figures show the extensive microvillus interactions (white arrows, a; large black arrow, b) between follicle cells (FC) and the growing oocyte (O) during early stages of oogenesis (prior to the deposition of the zona pellucida) in which numerous intra-ooplasmic projections of the follicle cells are evident (black arrows, a). Higher magnifications of the oocyte–follicle cell interface show interactions involving gap junctions and occasional desmosomes (small black arrow, b) indicating the complexity of communication between germ and somatic cell compartments at this stage of oogenesis

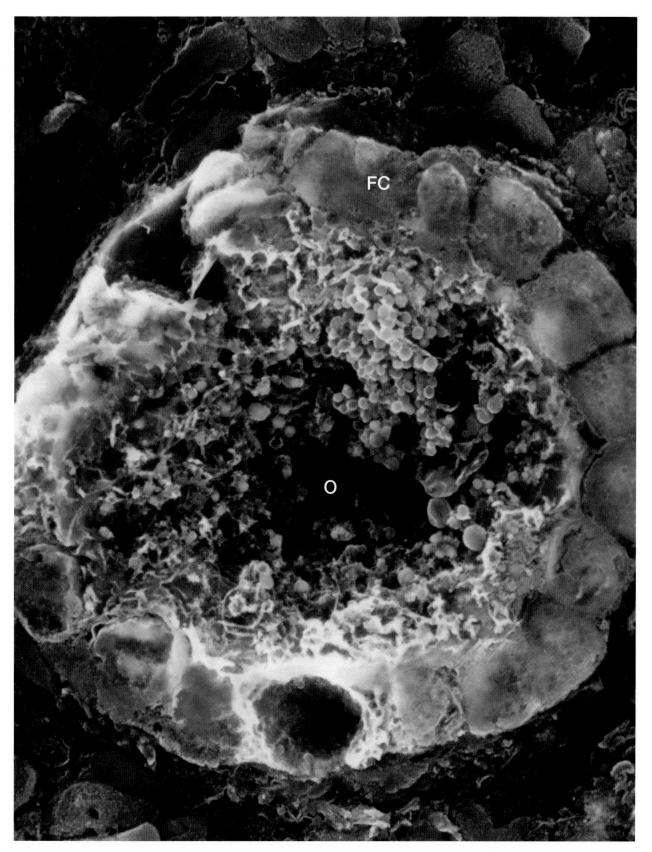

Figure 44   This SEM image of a primary follicle in an adult human ovary was obtained after partial digestion of the oocyte (O) to remove the nucleus and soluble components of the cytoplasm. The cuboidal/polyhedral follicle cells (FC) closely apposed to the oocyte are unaffected by this treatment. As shown in Figures 45–47, this method allows the organization and structure of organelles and cytoskeletal elements that are resistant to treatment to be visualized

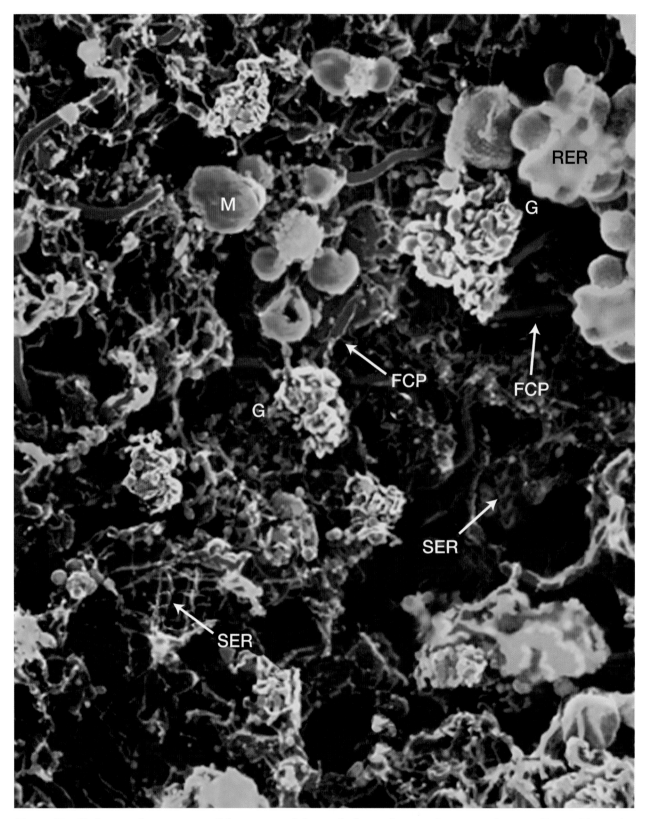

Figure 45 High-magnification views of the interior of the residual cytoplasm in the oocyte shown in Figure 44 reveal a complex structure in which long follicle cell projections (FCP) penetrate deeply into the oocyte and associate with Golgi complexes (G), mitochondria (M) and elements of the smooth (SER) and rough-surfaced endoplasmic reticulum (RER). These projections are thought to be conduits of bidirectional communication between the oocyte and its corresponding somatic cells and may function in early oogenesis to provide nutrients and regulatory factors and to remove catabolites produced by the oocyte

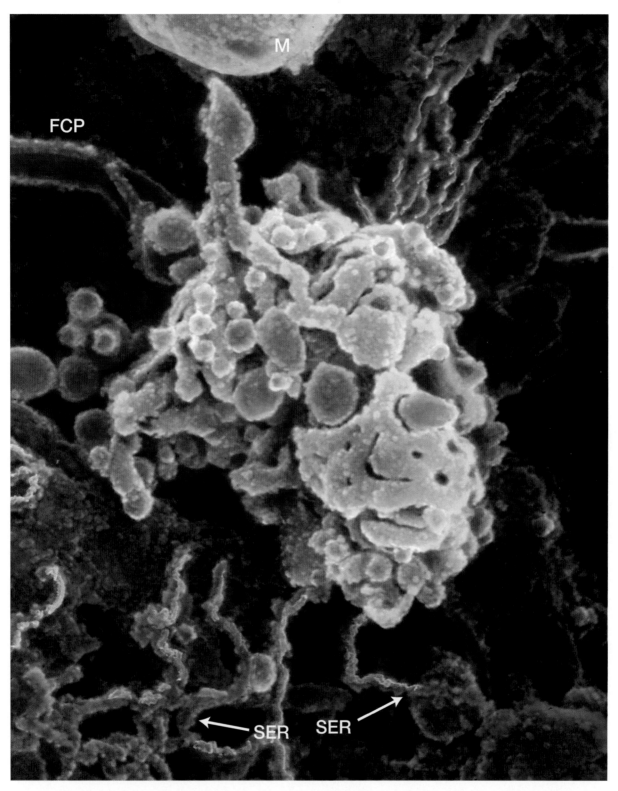

Figure 46 At increased magnification, the outermost cisternae of a Golgi complex are seen. The Golgi complex is formed by stacks of membranous saccules and vesicles that function in the post-translational modification of proteins, primarily those targeted for secretion or insertion into the plasma membrane. In this image, the association between this Golgi complex, a mitochondrion (M), elements of the smooth-surfaced endoplasmic reticulum (SER) and an intracytoplasmic follicle cell projection (FCP) is clearly evident. Owing to the function of the Golgi complex in protein modification and transport, it has been suggested that molecular signals produced by the oocyte may pass into the follicular cell process and influence the biosynthetic activities of these cells. This mechanism of bidirectional molecular communication may be essential in normal oogenesis and in the establishment of embryo developmental competence after fertilization

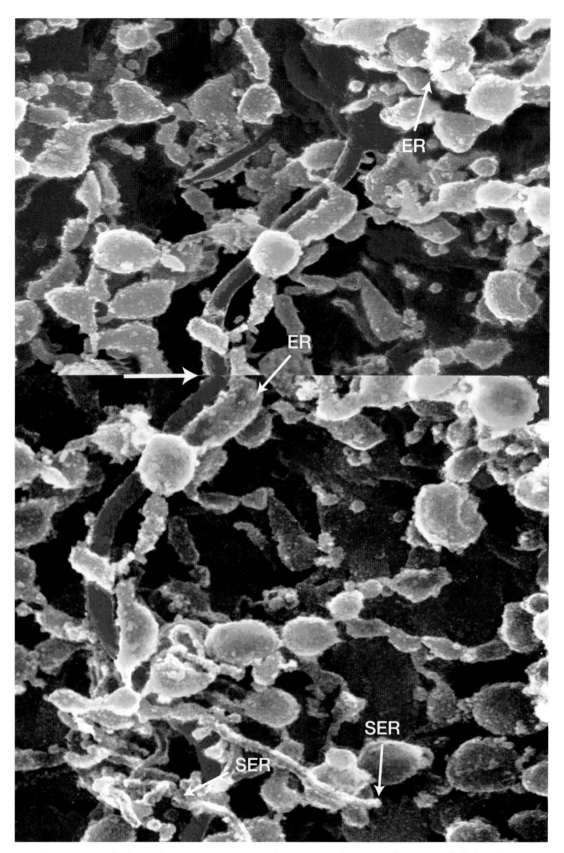

Figure 47 This composite high-resolution SEM image emphasizes the relationship between a follicle cell projection (large arrow) and elements of the endoplasmic reticulum (ER) in the cortical cytoplasm of the early oocyte. As with Golgi complexes, direct contact between the ER and a follicle cell projection may have regulatory functions in the coordinated development of the oocyte and follicle cells. SER, smoothed-surfaced endoplasmic reticulum

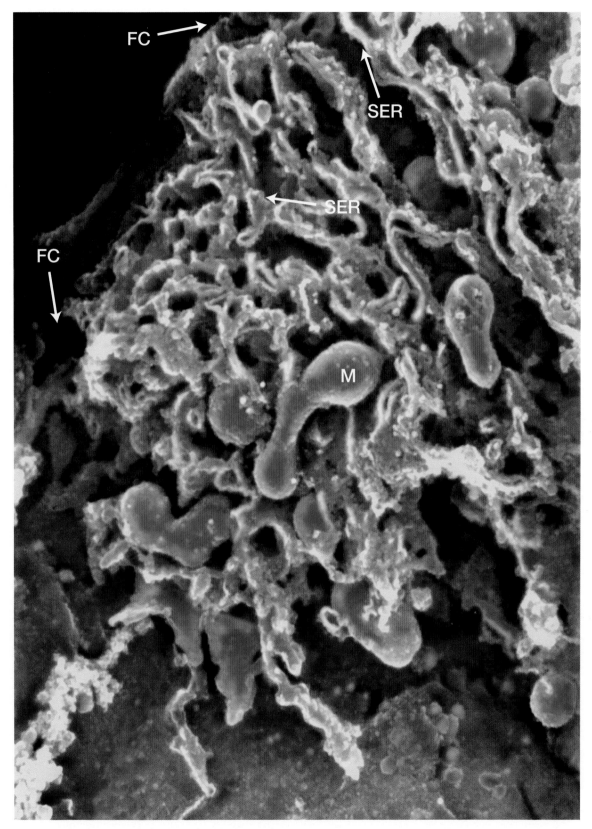

Figure 48 This SEM image demonstrates the association between mitochondria (M) and the smooth-surfaced endoplasmic reticulum (SER) in a follicle cell (FC) that sends projections into the developing oocyte. The association between fully developed mitochondria and the SER may be important in the regulation of mitochondrial respiration, which could upregulate levels of ATP production, and its transport into the oocyte by means of FCPs could provide an exogenous energy source for the oocyte

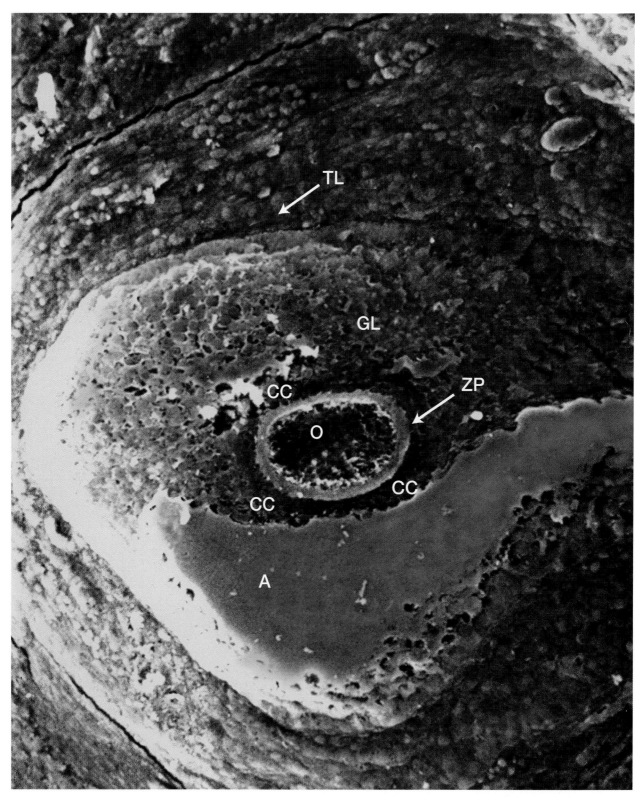

Figure 49 This SEM image shows the fractured surface of a developing antral follicle in an adult human ovary. The fully grown oocyte (O) surrounded by the zona pellucida (ZP) and a layer of cumulus–corona cells (CC) becomes eccentrically located within the follicle as fluid accumulation expands the antrum (A). Around the mural granulosa layer (GL) is the thecal layer (TL), through which capillaries course and, by serum transudation and diffusion, supply the developing follicle with oxygen

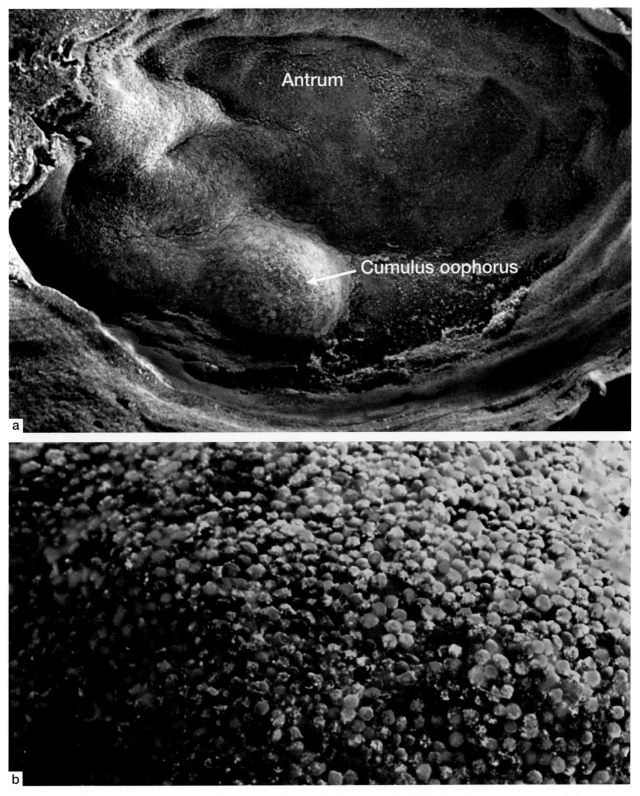

Figure 50 These SEM images reveal the internal details of a large antral follicle. In (a), the expansion of the antrum provides an unimpeded view of the cumulus oophorus that surrounds the oocyte. At higher magnification (b), the relatively uniform and spherical nature of the outermost granulosa cells of the cumulus oophorus is evident

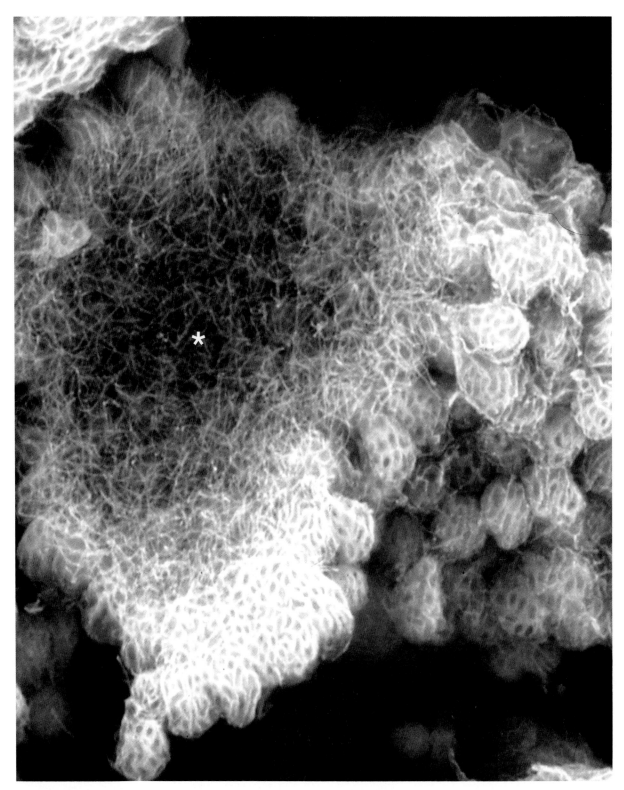

Figure 51 Changes in the nature of the interaction and communication between oocyte and corona–cumulus cells become critical during the preovulatory phase as they signal the final stages of oogenesis, leading to the resumption of meiosis and the final oocyte developmental processes required for fertilization. The innermost layer of the cumulus oophorus, the corona radiata, normally adheres to the zona pellucida and contacts the outer surface of the oocyte by means of transzonal projections. In this SEM image of a large antral follicle, the dissolution of the zona pellucida and oocyte by the ODO method permits the direct visualization of the transzonal follicle cell projections and affords a view of what the oocyte had 'seen' in the intact state. At relatively low magnification, the region formerly occupied by the oocyte (asterisk) occurs as a dense meshwork of slender follicle cell projections

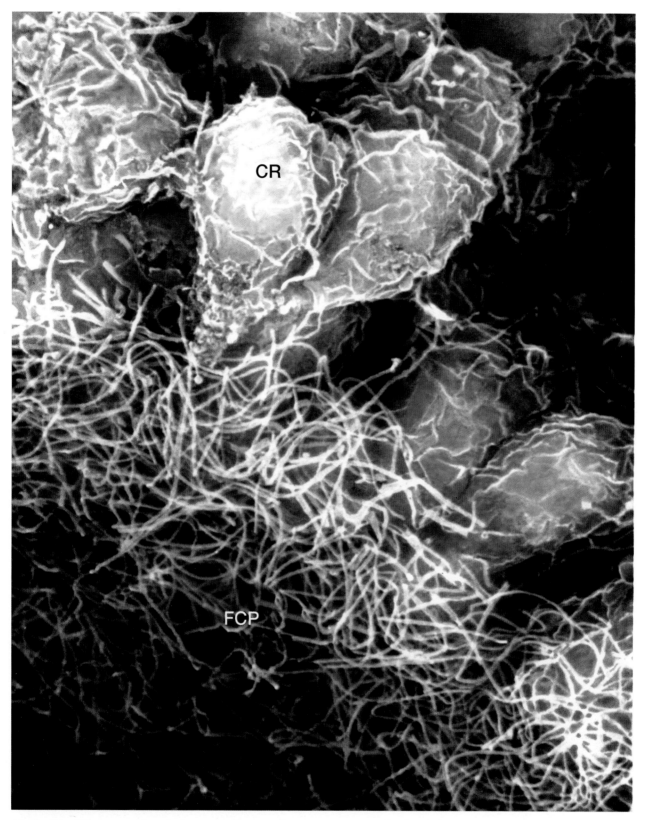

Figure 52 When viewed at higher magnification, the extensive network of cytoplasmic projections (FCP) that extends through the zona pellucida from the pear-shaped cells of the corona radiata (CR) is clearly evident. These and other follicular extensions contribute to a tremendous expansion of the surface area of corona cells, and their contact with the oocyte allows the structural basis for bidirectional movement of molecules and ions between the germ and somatic cell compartments

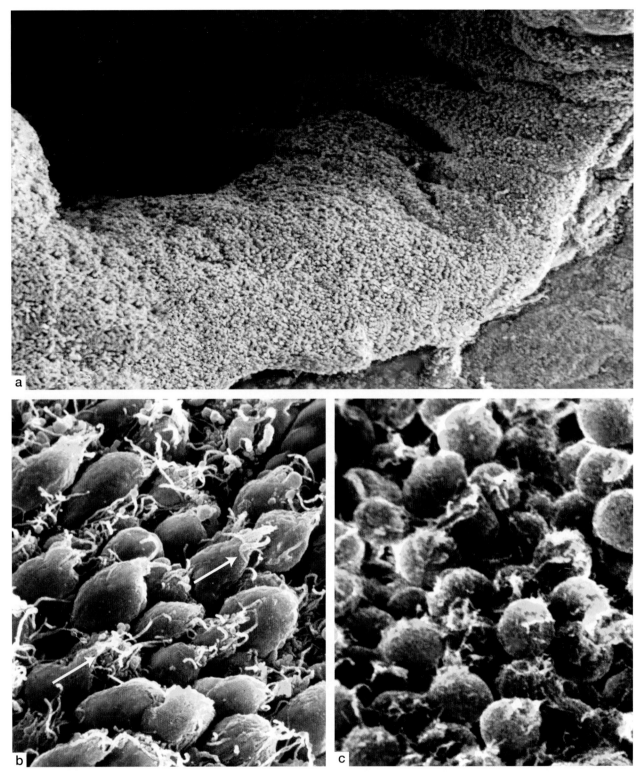

Figure 53   (a) is a low-magnification SEM image of a human preovulatory (Graafian) follicle that has been prepared to reveal internal details. With mechanical rupture of the follicle it is often possible to obtain samples of mural and cumulus granulosa for analytical purposes. (b) and (c) are SEM images of preovulatory mural and cumulus granulosa cells, respectively, from such a Graafian follicle. Many of the mural granulosa cells are oblong and have apical tufts of elongated microvilli (arrows) that distinguish them at the SEM level from their cumulus granulosa counterparts, which are usually spherical (c)

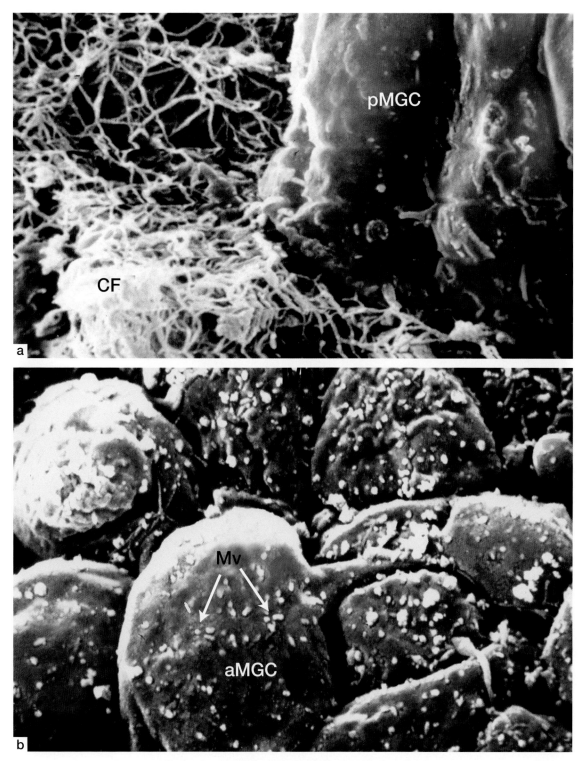

Figure 54 These figures are enlarged views of peripheral (pMGC, a) and antral mural granulosa cells (aMGC, b) in a human preovulatory follicle. Peripheral MGC appear as elongated steroid-secreting cells with a relatively smooth (microvillus-free) lateral surface adorned by scattered blebs that may reflect their secretory activity. These cells sit on a meshwork of collagen fibers (CF) that is part of the basement membrane associated with the follicular wall. This structure provides a wide area for bidirectional perifollicular traffic of nutrients, steroid precursors, oxygen, and growth and other regulatory factors. Antral MGC, like the majority of mural granulosa cells, develop pseudopodium-like processes and numerous cytoplasmic evaginations such as blebs and microvilli (Mv) on their surface

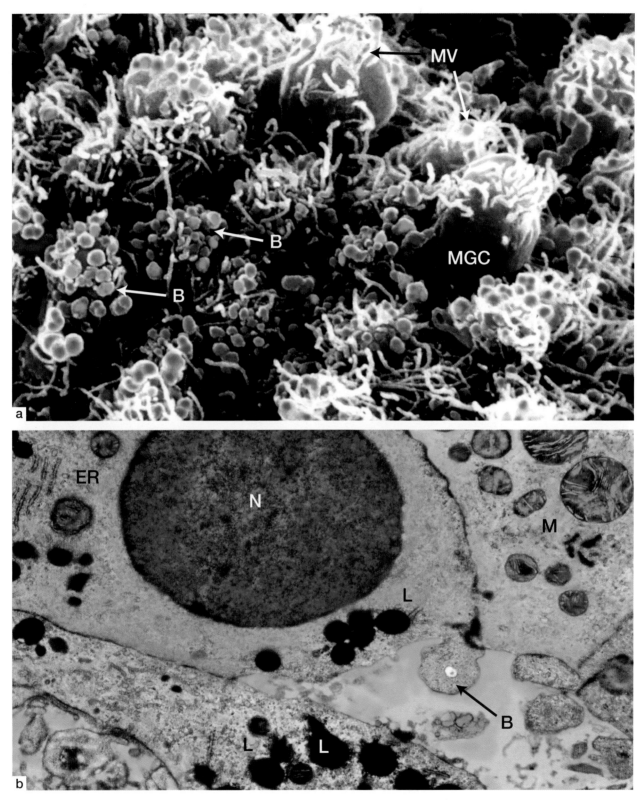

Figure 55 Just before ovulation, an increase in the density of LH receptors and a shift in steroid production from estrogen to progesterone are accompanied by dynamic changes in the surface architecture of mural granulosa cells (MGC) that, when viewed by SEM (a) show an increased number of secretory bleb-like structures (B) and long, slender microvilli (MV). The structure and organization of the cytoplasm as imaged by TEM is also complex (b), with networks of endoplasmic reticulum (ER), lipid droplets (L) and differentiated mitochondria with tubular cristae (M) indicative of cells active in steroidogenesis. Note the presence of a voluminous nucleus (N) and blebs (B) of various sizes

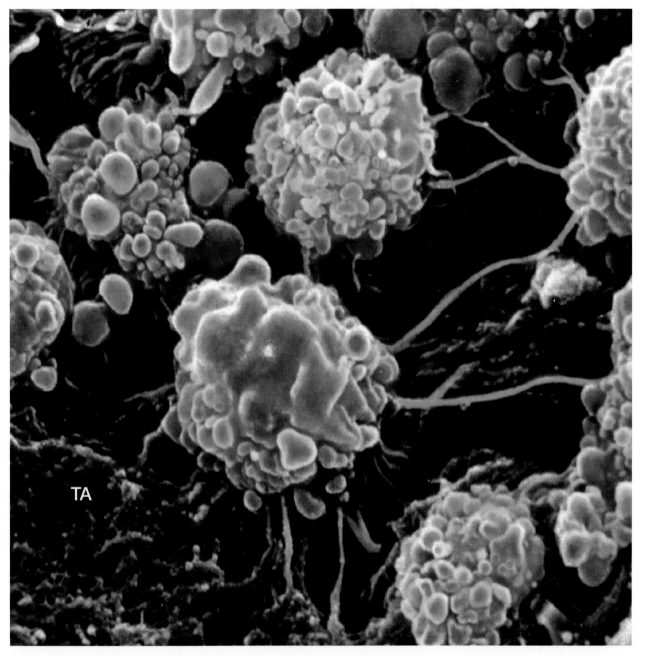

Figure 56 At the apex of the human preovulatory follicle, the superficial cells are uncoupled, possess a mulberry-like appearance, are connected by thin extensions and expose large open areas of the underlying tunica albuginea (TA). The appearance of these cells is suggestive of an apoptotic process by which apical cells degenerate and exfoliate before the follicle ruptures at ovulation

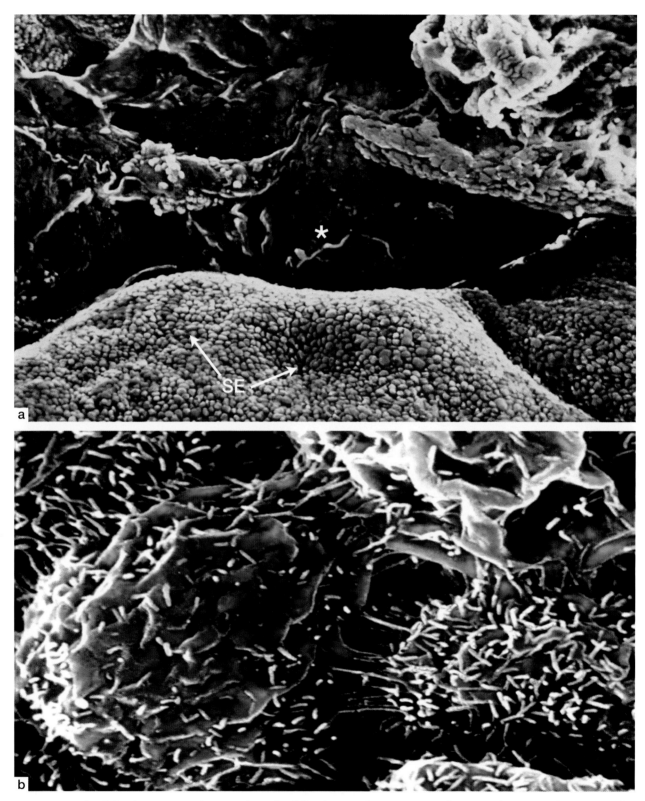

Figure 57 The follicular stigma is the site where the follicular membrane ruptures during ovulation and from which the mature oocyte–cumulus complex is expelled. This figure shows this region approximately 20 hours after ovulation when repair of the ruptured follicle begins as fluids and reactive tissues close the stigma (asterisk, a). The disrupted area is covered by numerous flattened cells which migrate from adjacent undamaged zones of the superficial epithelium (SE), as well as cells with numerous slender protrusions (filopodia and microvilli; b) which are indicative of active mitotic proliferation related to the regenerative process

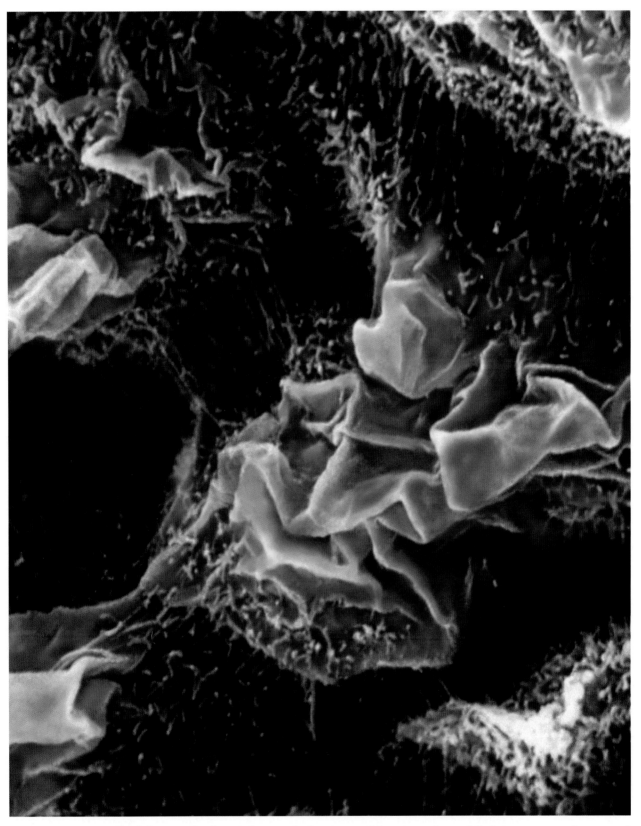

Figure 58 Many cells of the superficial epithelium at the basal area of the postovulatory follicle have an irregular size and shape with apical cellular protrusions and ruffles, indicative of secretory or endocytotic processes. These features may also represent an expansion of the plasma membrane surface that is a prelude to their becoming highly flattened and elongated as they migrate to the stigma and cover the follicular rupture

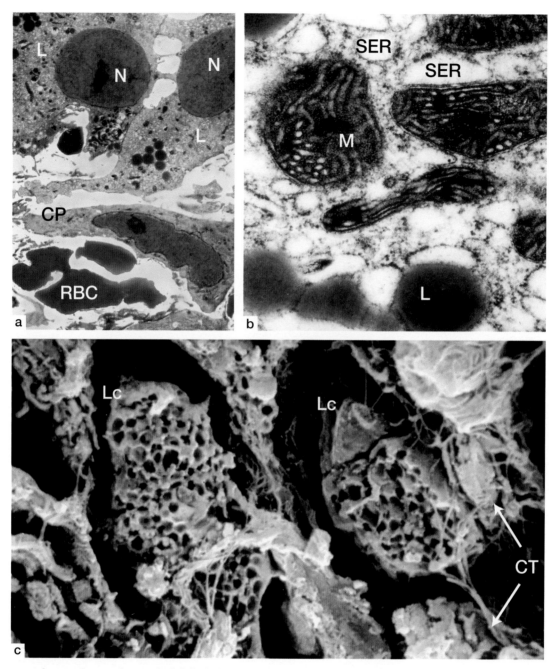

Figure 59 After ovulation, the residual follicle begins to transform into a steroid-secreting endocrine organ, the corpus luteum. The corpus luteum becomes a solid mass of closely packed, polyhedral luteal cells that are derived from both the mural granulosa and thecal layers which are organized on a matrix of connective tissue through which nascent blood vessels course. This organization is typical of an endocrine tissue that secretes progesterone, which is the central molecule involved in the establishment and maintenance of pregnancy. The life span of a corpus luteum is determined by whether or not pregnancy is established and persists normally. If the oocyte is fertilized and the embryo implants and continues through gestation, the corpus luteum enlarges and actively secretes for several months. If pregnancy has not been established, the corpus luteum undergoes luteolysis, a degenerative process required for a new cycle of follicular growth, development and ovulation to occur. (a, b) and (c) are TEM and SEM images, respectively, of progesterone-secreting granulosa–luteal cells in a developing corpus luteum on the 7th day of the luteal phase. Strands of connective tissue through which red blood cell (RBC)-containing capillaries (CP) course form a delicate network around groups of luteal cells and serve as a conduit for secreted progesterone (a). The luteal cells (Lc) enlarge, show voluminous nuclei (N) and become irregular in shape as they elaborate cytoplasmic extensions. Numerous large mitochondria with villiform cristae (M, b), smooth endoplasmic reticulum (SER) and numerous lipid droplets (L) are characteristic features of a mature granulosa–lutein cell. As observed by SEM, regressing luteal cells (Lc) surrounded by loose strands of connective tissue (CT) contain numerous lipid droplets that appear empty due to sample preparation, giving the luteal tissue a typical honeycomb-like appearance (c)

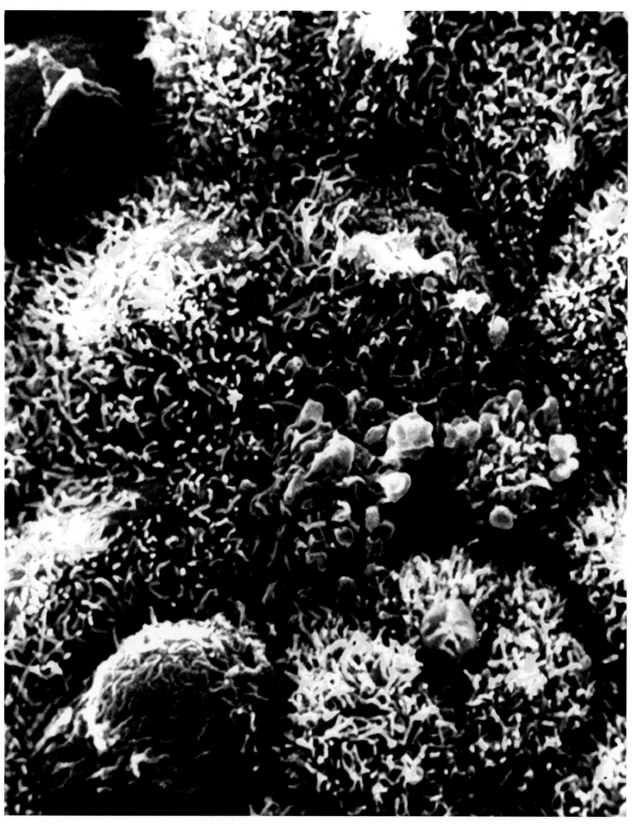

Figure 60　This SEM image of the surface of an ovary from a patient with polycystic ovarian disease (PCOD) demonstrates the atypical characteristics associated with anovulation. The entire surface of the ovary is covered by a highly proliferative superficial epithelium composed of tightly packed cells whose surface architecture is characterized by dense microvilli, solitary cilia, blebs, filopodia and ruffles. For PCOD patients, this atypical and unusually proliferative superficial epithelial layer may result from chronically high levels of luteinizing hormone (LH)

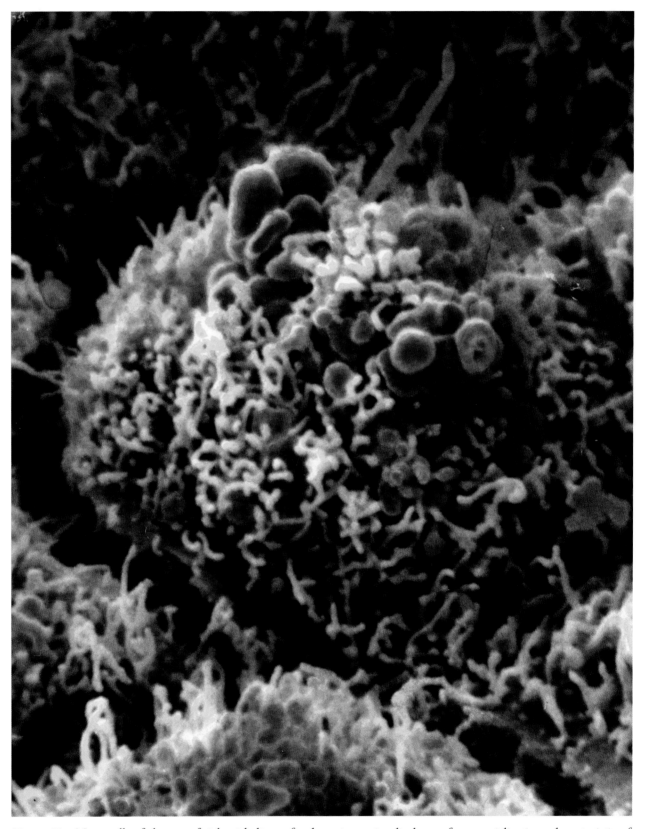

Figure 61 Many cells of the superficial epithelium of polycystic ovaries display surface specializations characteristic of rapidly dividing cells such as microvilli, blebs, ruffles and filopodia. This SEM image is representative of this type of cell common in cases of polycystic ovarian disease

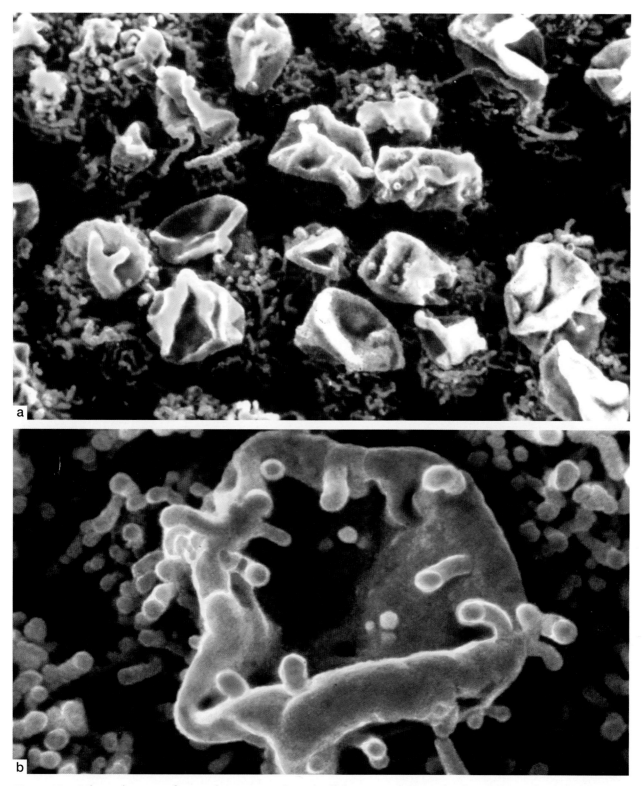

Figure 62 Other indications of atypical activities and rapid cell division in the superficial epithelium of polycystic ovaries are shown in these figures. Extensive ruffling of the plasma membrane (a) is a feature common to rapidly growing cells and the surface protrusions that emerge from the ruffled membrane (b) may be related to endocytotic processes whereby cells take up substances without passing them through cell membrane receptor-mediated process

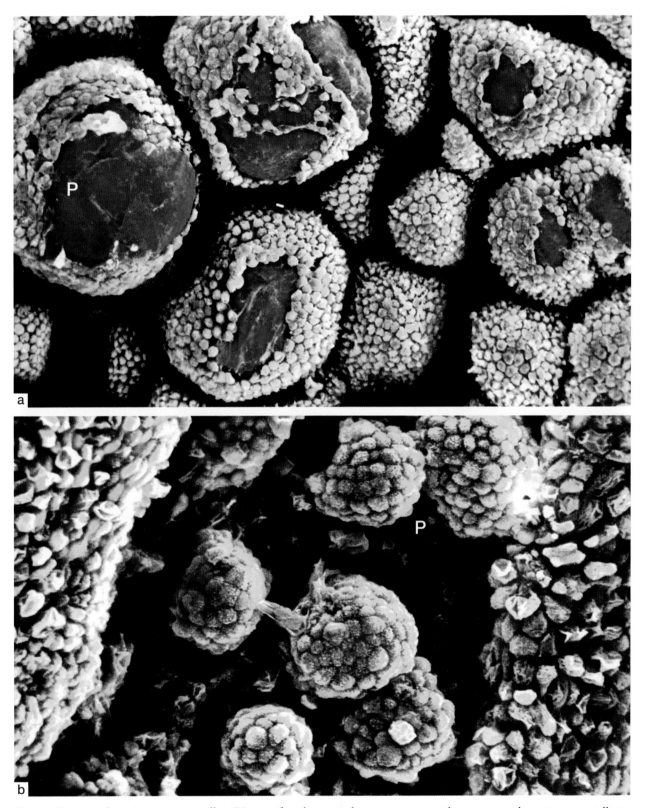

Figure 63 In polycystic ovaries, papillae (P) are often larger and more numerous than in normal ovaries, especially in advanced stages of development of the disease (a). Extensive papilla development in polycystic ovaries appears to be a continual process related to hormonal levels, and groups of papillae in early stages of formation can be seen throughout the ovarian surface (b). Unlike their more advanced counterparts, these papillae are completely covered by the superficial epithelium

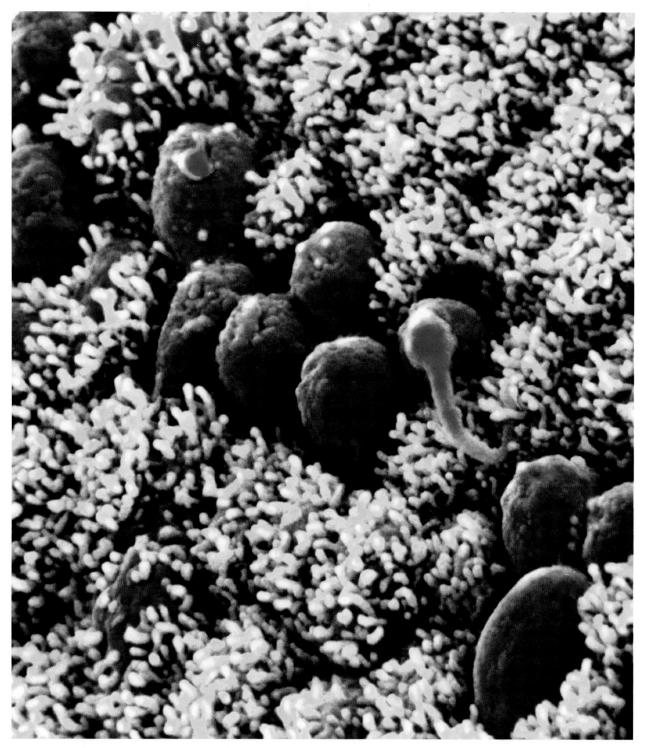

Figure 64 The occurrence of luteinized albeit unruptured follicles is common in anovulatory women. In cases of luteinized unruptured follicle (LUF) syndrome, the superficial cells express a dense population of microvilli and regions of cells with completely smooth surfaces are observed. The smooth-surfaced cells are an atypical feature that is characteristic of this anovulatory condition

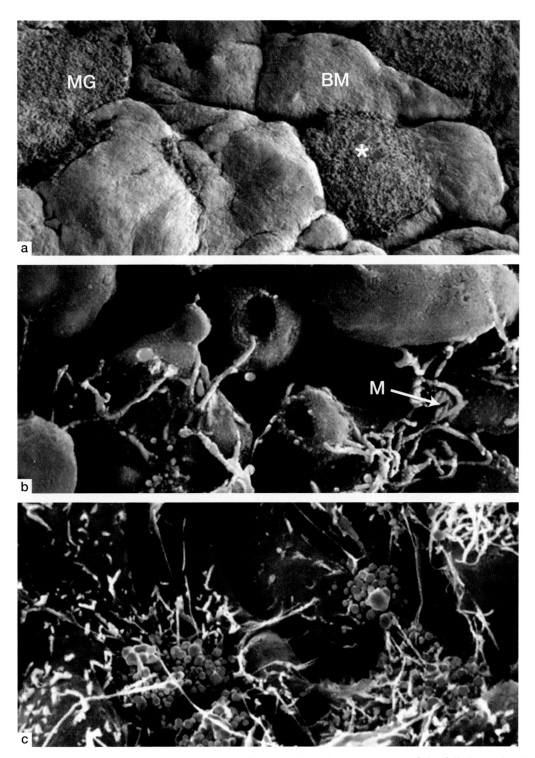

Figure 65 Pathology associated with polycystic ovaries also extends to the organization of the follicle. In the SEM image shown in (a), the mural granulosa (MG) that normally covers the follicular wall occurs in polycystic follicles as scattered areas of cells (asterisk) with large portions of the basement membrane (BM) exposed. This truncated granulosa layer rapidly degenerates. In advanced stages of this disease, mural granulosa cells show a completely different appearance, as they are smooth-surfaced, flattened, irregular in size and shape, and virtually devoid of any surface specializations indicative of secretory activity, displaying only a few distorted microvilli (M) and rare blebs (b). Even in the most advanced and longstanding cases of polycystic ovarian disease, some small patches of mural granulosa cells occur that exhibit surface features consistent with progesterone production. In contrast to what is shown in (b), these cells display long, slender microvilli, blebs and cytoplasmic extensions that in the normal postovulatory follicle are typical of luteinized cells (c)

Development of the mature oocyte and preimplantation-stage embryo

The dual engines of discovery and technology drive rapid developments in modern biology. The decoding of the human genome, the development of micro-array and proteomic technologies, and their application in molecular studies in a wide variety of experimental systems have facilitated our understanding of how individual genes or gene families function. This research enterprise has led to the mapping of molecular pathways that regulate normal activities or produce pathological conditions in multiple species ranging from insects to mammals, including the human. New findings continue to reveal pathways common among cells that define the basic 'principles of life' – those biochemical pathways and states of cytoplasmic organization that govern how all cells function and behave. These discoveries have become the foundation of modern molecular medicine, are the cornerstone of current research that seeks to identify specific genes or proteins whose expression patterns can be correlated with the type and severity of a disease, and thus lead to the development of treatments that use targeted drugs or other novel therapies.

The same experimental approach has been used to investigate what must be the single most important activity in which organisms are engaged: their reproduction. For mammals in general and the human in particular, early research has focused on identification of genes and signaling pathways which may be critical in the generation of developmentally competent gametes and embryos, and normal reproductive tract functions that are consistent with implantation and gestation to term[1,2]. Because molecular and biochemical activities often involve complex morphodynamic processes, a renewed interest in the fundamental structural and organizational

information afforded by SEM and TEM techniques has emerged with respect to reproductive tract tissues and embryonic cells. This type of analysis has been especially useful in the study of human oocytes and embryos generated in infertility treatments such as *in vitro* fertilization (IVF). In the case of IVF, certain types of common subcellular defects identified in oocytes have been associated with abnormal or arrested embryonic development[3]. Consequently, this section is largely devoted to recent SEM and TEM findings that pertain to normal and abnormal development in the mature human oocyte (Chapter 3) and preimplantation-stage embryo (Chapter 4).

HISTORICAL PERSPECTIVES ON THE ORIGIN OF THE EMBRYO

Few readers of this Atlas would question the fundamental principle of mammalian reproduction: namely, that an embryo develops from an oocyte that has been fertilized by a spermatozoon. Yet, while the natural origin of the embryo is a generally accepted fact, the current issue of when life 'begins'[4] has engendered levels of contentious public debate and discourse reminiscent of the major reproductive question of past centuries, which was whether the embryo developed from the male or female gamete. For example, embryologists of the 17th and 18th centuries were largely divided between two conflicting theories of sexual reproduction: the 'Animal-cultists', who believed that spermatozoa were the true germ cells, and the 'Ovulists,' who adhered to the supremacy of the female germ cell and the notion *ex ovo omnia*, or from the egg all. It was not until the advent of 'modern embryology' in the 19th century, beginning with von Baer's discovery in 1827[5] that the mammalian gamete, or oocyte, is contained within an ovarian cyst-like structure, the Graafian follicle, that a biparental origin of reproduction became a viable notion. The term Graafian follicle, used to this day, is named for Renier de Graaf who, in 1672, was the first (but not the only one of his contemporaries) to describe the egg-producing function of the ovary in his book *De mulierum organis generationi inservientibus tractatus novus*. Nevertheless, it was not until nearly 200 years after the publication of this treatise that van Beneden[6] and Hertwig[7] showed that both oocyte and sperm were required for fertilization in the mammal. With the realization that a child develops from a fertilized ovum, Haeckel[8] termed this one-cell structure a 'stem-cell' or *cytula*, because its properties were uniquely different from the female gamete, being as it were, 'the product or resultant of the paternal life-movement that is conveyed in the spermatozoon and the maternal life-movement that is contributed by the ovum.' By the end of the 19th century, debates concerning the true origin of the embryo largely ended as the notion of biparental reproduction became established doctrine. How this doctrine was understood is perhaps best presented in the following passage from Haeckel:

> 'The process of fertilization by sexual conception consists essentially in the coalescence and fusing together of two different cells. The spermatozoon travels towards the ovum by it serpentine movements, and bores it way into the female cell. The nuclei of both sexual cells, attracted by a certain "affinity," approach each other and melt into one.'

The growing certainty with which different aspects of early development were viewed and understood in a biological context is what makes the narratives of previous generations of scientists so interesting. However, at the dawn of the 21st century new experimental findings may force a reconsideration of some of the most basic biological tenets of reproduction, including the central question of when life begins. Consider for example the following: (1) the production of viable offspring by somatic cell nuclear transfer, also known as cloning[9], (2) the birth of mice from embryos created by parthenogenetic (no sperm) activation of genetically modified oocytes[10] and (3) the generation of embryonic germ cells and apparently competent male and female

gametes from embryonic stem cells grown entirely *in vitro*, i.e. without an organized ovarian or testicular contribution[11,12]. Contemporary clinical embryology and the technologies used in reproductive medicine have also created important issues that are as contentious today as were the seemingly arcane topics of debate between Animalcultists and Ovulists 300 years ago. For example, today we ask (1) whether an embryo has legal rights and, if so, at what stage after sperm penetration should they apply; (2) should such rights be applied equally to embryos produced by cloning or by natural fertilization; (3) should specialized insemination techniques be permitted in infertility treatments with sperm carrying known and inheritable genetic defects, including those which will result in infertile male offspring[13]; (4) is it medically ethical for oocytes to be subjected to invasive manipulations and novel cellular therapies in order to be 'rescued' from presumed developmental failure[14]; or (5) should IVF and chromosomal analysis of early embryos be used to enable gender selection (so-called 'family-balancing') for both fertile and infertile women, rather than for the detection of known or suspected genetic defects and mutations, for which the technique of preimplantation genetic diagnosis was originally intended[15]? These questions are not simply of academic interest but have important practical implications as well. How different societies reconcile conflicting opinions within their populations and whether they are able to derive a workable consensus will determine for each, permissible basic research (e.g. embryonic stem cell derivation from cloned embryos) and clinical practices in assisted reproduction centers (e.g. gender selection).

THE ROLE OF ELECTRON MICROSCOPY IN CLINICAL IN VITRO FERTILIZATION

While the above questions are important topics for debate, two facts concerning human reproduction are not debatable: most fertilized human embryos are developmentally incompetent; and developmental incompetence largely originates in the oocyte prior to fertilization[16,17]. That high frequencies of early developmental failure (embryo wastage) occur in the human has been clearly demonstrated over the past 25 years when outcome results from clinical IVF are calculated on a per embryo basis[18]. Likewise, the notion that early embryo wastage largely originates from oocyte defects has been confirmed by cytological and genetic analysis of thousands of oocytes and developmentally arrested embryos produced for or by IVF, respectively[3,15]. Most of our current knowledge about the structural biology of the human oocyte and the progression of preimplantation embryogenesis from fertilization through the hatched blastocyst stage comes from residual oocytes and embryos donated to research by patients who underwent treatment in IVF-related centers. In this respect, electron microscopy has been particularly useful in analyzing the fine structural details of cytoplasmic defects or disorders seen at the light microscopic level and which have been associated with poor or reduced developmental competence[3,19,20]. All current schemes used to assess human oocyte and embryo competence by non-invasive methods include some type of subjective light microscopic observations of cell and cytoplasmic characteristics[20,21]. Recently, computer-based algorithms and digitalization of light microscopic images have added objective (i.e. quantifiable) criteria such as cell shape and volume to these assessments[22]. The potential for TEM and SEM to increase the sensitivity of oocyte or embryo evaluations is based on the ability to resolve subtle differences in cytoplasmic organization that may have or be associated with negative developmental consequences. In this regard, many of the fine structural images presented in this section describe subcellular conditions that could have adverse downstream consequences. Once identified in the fixed state, the development of methods for their detection in the living state may go a long way in improving oocyte and embryo competence assessments in clinical IVF.

It seems likely that, for the near future, treatment of the infertile patient will continue to require oocytes derived from ovarian follicles and embryos that result from fertilization with a spermatozoon. The SEM and TEM micrographs we present have direct relevance to infertility treatments as they demonstrate what may be considered both normal and abnormal patterns of early human development that have been observed in actual IVF cycles. Likewise, because ovarian follicles are the primary targets of current endocrine treatments that produce multiple oocytes for insemination, an understanding of how the intrafollicular environment may influence oocyte competence[17] is aided by viewing the fine structural context in which the oocyte coexists with follicular cells, especially under changing hormonal conditions such as those described in Chapter 2. Most of the electron microscopic images in this section have been artificially colored. As with the previous section and an earlier Atlas related to menopausal aging[23], this was done for esthetic reasons and because differential coloration of specific tissues, cell types, organelles and other subcellular elements enables the reader to obtain a more immediate and incisive view of cellular structure, organization and intercellular relationships than afforded in the original grayscale images. The application of new technologies and gene discoveries in reproductive medicine and biology will identify molecular or genetic defects associated with infertility or reproductive tract pathology. The development of treatments for such disorders will require an understanding of the cellular defects in affected tissues and cells, and it is our hope that the fine structural images presented in this Atlas contribute to these research and clinical efforts.

3   Preovulatory maturation of the human oocyte

CLINICAL ASPECTS

During each natural menstrual cycle, multiple small follicles enter the ovulatory pathway and, over a relatively short period of time, several may grow in response to follicle stimulating hormone (FSH). However, one follicle typically becomes dominant (the so-called 'dominant follicle') and develops competency to ovulate a fully grown oocyte in response to luteinizing hormone (LH), a pituitary gonadotropin whose sudden discharge is termed the 'LH surge' owing to the rapid increase of circulating levels of this protein hormone. For certain infertility treatments, especially those involving IVF, the principal aim of the endocrine management of the menstrual cycle is to increase systemic levels of FSH in order to promote the development of multiple dominant follicles. Collectively, the various clinical protocols used to manage the female cycle are referred to as controlled ovarian hyperstimulation (COHS). The ideal endpoint of COHS is the production of a cohort of fully grown and developmentally competent oocytes that have simultaneously resumed meiosis in response to an ovulatory dose of LH, or its functional equivalent: human chorionic gonadotropin (hCG). The preovulatory maturation of the oocyte is usually described in terms of a coordinated series of stage-specific changes at the nuclear (nuclear maturation) and cytoplasmic (cytoplasmic maturation) levels that culminate in the ovulation of a fertilizable gamete[24].

Nuclear maturation encompasses all events associated with chromatin condensation into bivalent chromosomes and completion of the first reductional division of meiosis followed by the imposition of a second meiotic arrest at metaphase II. Shortly before ovulation, a grossly asymmetrical cell division produces a diploid oocyte and a 'mini-cell', the first polar body, whose formation begins as an evagination of the oolemma and ooplasm directly above the metaphase I spindle, which is usually located in the subplasmalemmal cytoplasm. The presence of outwardly segregating mass chromosomes promotes the formation of this evagination[25,26] and, within minutes, this protrusion, containing a relatively minute amount of ooplasm and a complete diploid set of chromosomes, separates from the oocyte proper. Most of the numerical chromosomal disorders (aneuploidies) that occur at high frequency in newly ovulated metaphase II human oocytes and which are passed on to the embryo after fertilization arise during meiosis I, and result from defects in the process of chromosomal segregation[27–29]. Genomic imprinting can now be added to the list of processes associated with nuclear maturation owing to the finding that this critical genetic modification is completed shortly before ovulation[30]. Genomic imprinting (gene silencing) involves enzymatic molecular modification (methylation) of a small number of genes in order to inhibit their expression (transcription). Silencing of these specific genes occurs differentially in sperm and oocytes such that transcription is from either the maternal or the paternal allele. This pattern of uniparental gene expression is established in the embryo and persists in the somatic cells of the individual throughout life. Certain imprinted genes have important regulatory functions that control rates of cell division and tissue/organ growth[31]. In these instances biallelic expression (i.e. both maternal and paternal copies) could have adverse developmental effects. For example, biallelic expression has been suggested to be the cause of a common pattern of abnormal intrauterine development occasionally observed in certain animal systems (sheep, cow) in which oocyte maturation, fertilization or preimplantation embryogenesis occurred entirely *in vitro* and where, after embryo transfer to suitably prepared recipients, fetal development was characterized by extreme overgrowth[32]. It is thought that fertilization *in vitro* prior to the completion of oocyte genomic imprinting or, in other cases, the prolongation of early embryogenesis under suboptimal culture conditions, or both, may promote differential biallelic expression of growth-regulating genes that appear to be responsible for this syndrome[33]. Nevertheless it is noteworthy that, in over 25 years of clinical IVF with COHS and millions of oocytes inseminated and embryos transferred, extreme fetal overgrowth of this type has not been evident in the over 2 million babies born to date. However, there is growing concern[34] that the design of current culture media used in clinical IVF and certain clinical practices, such as *in vitro* oocyte growth and maturation, and the extension of embryo culture to the hatched blastocyst stage, may adversely affect DNA methylation patterns[35] leading to a potential increase in the occurrence of rare genetic defects such as retinoblastoma, that result from gene-specific imprinting disorders[36].

Cytoplasmic maturation involves a progressive series of dynamic structural and molecular changes that are coordinated in the ooplasm and oolemma in space and time that collectively (1) prepare the oocyte for sperm penetration, (2) increase the likelihood that penetration will be monospermic and, after penetration, (3) enable the sequential expression of developmental processes associated with fertilization and early embryogenesis. For the purpose of *in vitro* fertilization in the human, cytoplasmic maturation is considered to be initiated with the gonadotropin-induced resumption of meiosis at the GV stage and, for successful monospermic fertilization, should be completed at or shortly after ovulation[37,38]. Results from animal studies that are relevant for the human indicate that defects in the normal sequence of cytoplasmic maturation can have negative consequences for embryogenesis. For example, errors in cytoplasmic maturation have been correlated with abnormalities in cell division and slow rates of cell division that result in embryos which are stage-inappropriate with respect to cell number, arrest during cleavage or fail to implant[39].

Over a quarter of a century's experience with clinical IVF provides abundant support for the notion that defects in preovulatory oocyte maturation are responsible for certain types of fertilization failures, are largely responsible for the high frequency of early embryo demise seen during the preimplantation stages and may have adverse developmental consequences that are not evident until after implantation[40]. These defects may be especially relevant causes of developmental failure for human oocytes where cytoplasmic and nuclear maturation occur *in vitro*[40]. Experimental and clinical research studies designed to understand the etiology and developmental consequences of maturational defects have found that certain intrafollicular conditions, especially if they occur during the latter stages of follicular growth and the LH/hCG-induced preovulatory period, can have adverse downstream consequences for human embryogenesis during the preimplantation stages. For example, high-resolution Doppler ultrasonographic methods have been used to quantify and characterize perifollicular blood flow rates and patterns, respectively, in natural menstrual cycles and cycles of COHS[41–43]. The results demonstrate that, within cohorts of fully grown (Graafian) follicles, including those in the same ovary, the rate of perifollicular blood flow is follicle-specific and appears to be related to the post-fertilization developmental competence of the corresponding oocyte. These studies indicate that grossly normal-appearing metaphase II oocytes derived from fully grown follicles with poor or undetectable perifollicular blood flow tend to have higher frequencies of aneuploidy and, after fertilization, a reduced potential to develop progressively and normally. In contrast, so-called 'top quality' embryos with high implantation and ongoing pregnancy potential have been correlated with oocytes obtained from 'high-flow' follicles[43–46]. It has been proposed that follicle-specific differences in perifollicular blood flow rates (high-to-undetectable) and characteristics (proportion of follicle with detectable blood flow) reflect corresponding differences in the degree of expansion of the perifollicular capillary bed which in turn may be related to the ability of the underlying follicle to produce and secrete potent angiogenesis-promoting growth factors[46]. Gaulden[47] was the first to suggest that poor perifollicular vascularity could be associated with severe intrafollicular hypoxia and, if so, contribute to the genesis of chromosomal aneuploidies if such a condition altered the physiology of the oocyte cytoplasm during preovulatory maturation. Although untested, her hypothesis suggests that underoxygenation of follicular fluid associated with inadequate perifollicular blood flow has eventual metabolic consequences for the oocyte. These result in a slight reduction of intracellular pH to levels that begin to compromise the normality of the microtubular component of the metaphase spindle(s). According to this notion, chromosomal segregation disorders such as trisomy-producing non-disjunction (e.g. trisomy 21 or Down syndrome) would tend to occur at significantly high frequencies in oocytes that matured in undervascularized and underoxygenated follicles, and would be of particular relevance in women of advanced reproductive age, because this condition increasingly affects the Graafian follicles they produce.

Much of what we know about the fine structure of human oocytes comes from a wide variety of oocytes obtained from women of different ages and etiologies of infertility undergoing IVF treatment. Human oocytes available for light or electron microscopic evaluation tend to be those which are meiotically immature, mature oocytes that fail to fertilize after insemination *in vitro*, or those which exhibit obvious cytoplasmic defects that may preclude their use in IVF attempts. For the TEM images described below, many were obtained from mature oocytes that were donated to research and judged normal by light microscopy. Images of oocytes obtained from follicles with known differences in perifollicular circulation or intrafollicular biochemistry currently thought to be related to developmental competence are absent from this collection. However, the images present details of normal differences in fine structure that may be useful in future studies that examine oocytes obtained from follicles in which intrafollicular conditions are known to be suboptimal for or inconsistent with normal developmental competence. Because preovulatory maturation in all mammals begins with oocytes arrested at the germinal vesicle stage, the following describes the reinitiation of arrested meiosis in the human that begins at this stage.

THE GERMINAL VESICLE STAGE OF THE HUMAN OOCYTE

Preovulatory maturation of the oocyte is initiated spontaneously with the LH surge or is induced during infertility treatments by the administration of hCG or recombinant LH in cycles of COHS. The reinitiation of meiosis, which had been arrested in prophase of meiosis I since the fetal stages of oogenesis, is generally thought to 'begin' with the cessation of gap junction-mediated intercellular communication between the oocyte and the somatic granulosa cells of the corona radiata and cumulus oophorus. Meiotic arrest at the germinal vesicle (GV) stage is maintained by relatively high intracytoplasmic levels of certain small regulatory molecules such as cyclic AMP (cAMP), which, in the case of this molecule, is maintained by balancing its catabolism with endogenous (oocyte) synthesis and uptake from the surrounding somatic cells. High intracytoplasmic levels of cAMP in the immature mammalian oocyte maintain meiotic arrest by inhibiting the activity of certain proteins in the 'maturation promotion factor' complex that regulate the cell cycle. The LH surge is associated with an abrupt drop in ooplasmic cAMP that terminates the longstanding inhibition on meiotic progression as cell cycle-related processes are activated. It is generally thought that the LH surge causes a sudden retraction of FSH-sensitized (follicle cell) transzonal processes from the oolemma that is followed within the ooplasm by a sharp drop in cAMP[48].

LH-induced meiotic 'reactivation' usually involves fully grown oocytes contained in fully grown follicles (Graafian follicles) that under FSH stimulation have developed a well-expanded fluid-filled antrum, a robust mural granulosa that is actively engaged in estrogen biosynthesis, and cumulus and corona granulosa cells that are sensitive to LH. In order to visualize the oocyte directly, the surrounding layers of somatic coronal and cumulus cells are removed by enzymatic or mechanical means, revealing a seemingly uncomplicated cell that is the largest cell in the human body. The fully grown human GV-stage oocyte was noted in 19th century descriptions [e.g. reference 8] as a unique cell, owing to its size (nearly 0.1 mm or 100 μm in diameter), enclosure by a clear 'glass-like shell' or zona pellucida, and presence of a large nucleus, or germinal vesicle, containing a prominent spherical nucleolus (Figure 66a). Although rare, binucleated human oocytes have been observed in follicular aspirates obtained for IVF. However, binucleation is not the artifactual result of COHS because it is also evident *in situ* when standard histological (i.e. light microscopic) sections taken at different levels through surgical specimens have included preantral and antral (Graafian) follicles (Figure 66b, c). While the origin of this lethal defect is unclear, it is commonly believed that fusion of two oocytes during early oogenesis is the most likely etiology. In the binucleate oocyte shown, a distinct nucleolus is present in one nucleus while scattered chromatin is evident in the other, suggesting that two different states of nuclear organization may coexist in these unusual gametes. In clinical IVF, fully grown GV-stage oocytes are often aspirated after ovulation induction from fully grown (FSH-stimulated) follicles. Their occurrence suggests that the oocyte or its surrounding somatic (cumulus oophorus and corona radiata) cells, or both, may have been unable to respond to intrafollicular conditions that promote preovulatory maturation, or that such conditions failed to develop in these follicles.

TEM studies show comparable states of cytoplasmic and nuclear organization in human GV-stage oocytes obtained from fully grown antral follicles after COHS and those mechanically extracted from preantral or early antral follicles in surgical specimens obtained after oophorectomy. Similar to the ovulated metaphase II oocyte, the GV-stage oocyte is surrounded by a mass of follicle/granulosa cells (Figure 67) composed of two basic compartments: an innermost layer, the corona radiata that rests upon the zona pellucida and communicates directly with the oocyte by means of transzonal processes (see Chapter 2; TZP, Figure 68); and an outer layer, termed the cumulus oophorus. The so-called cumulus layer is particularly important in the fertilization process because it is at this cellular boundary that sperm undergo the acrosome reaction resulting in the release of the enzyme hyaluronidase which digests the hyaluronic acid matrix between cumulus cells. Because of this enzymatic release, motile sperm progressively pass between cumulus granulosa cells to reach the zona surface. Molecular signaling and communication between oocyte and somatic cell compartments largely involve the transzonal process (TZP, Figure 69a) that originates from hundreds of circumferentially located coronal cells. Contact between the 'foot' of the TZP and the oolemma involves gap junctions (Figure 69b). It is now clear from experimental studies that a variety of potent growth factors and other signaling molecules produced by the oocyte probably pass through these processes and participate in the regulation of granulosa cell proliferation and differentiation during follicular growth and development[49,50]. Molecular signals passing into the oocyte from cumulus and coronal cells regulate the meiotic status of the oocyte and reinitiate the cell cycle prior to ovulation. Loss of functional intercellular communication may be one factor responsible for the occurrence of GV-stage oocytes in aspirates of fully expanded follicles during IVF cycles that involved COHS.

Fine structural analysis of the interface between oocyte and transzonal processes has been especially useful in understanding possible mechanisms of intercellular communication within the developing human follicle. Transzonal processes contain dense linear arrays of microtubules and microfilaments in which cytoplasmic components such as SER, mitochondria and vacuoles are located. The microtubular arrays appear to form the structural basis for bidirectional transport of regulatory molecules between oocyte and granulosa cells, and the detection of mitochondria in the transzonal processes suggests a possible exogenous source of ATP that can pass into the oocyte through gap junctions[51]. The presence of numerous small vesicles in both the cytoplasm of the transzonal process where it contacts the oolemma and in corresponding subplasmalemmal cytoplasm of the oocyte (i.e. subjacent to the site of process attachment) is a characteristic feature of this interface. These structures are indicated by black arrows in Figure 69b and may represent vesicular traffic between somatic and germ cell compartments that involves an endocytotic/exocytotic process. Comparatively large vacuoles and cisternae are common in the terminal portion of the transzonal elements (asterisks, Figure 69b) of the fully grown GV-stage human oocyte and may be a source of molecules that are transferred to the oocyte. During earlier stages of oogenesis, endocytosis may be an important mechanism by which maternally derived molecules and proteins released from coronal cells are taken up by the oocyte[52].

TEM analysis often shows differences in the density and distribution of cytoplasmic components in GV-stage oocytes aspirated from fully grown follicles after ovulation induction. Whether these differences are meaningful with respect to how normal developmental competence is established during oogenesis is a current focus of research in the field of clinical IVF. For example, the GV-stage oocyte shown in Figure 70 represents a common subcellular 'phenotype' in which large regions of the cytoplasm are devoid of organelles such as mitochondria, and in the subplasmalemmal cytoplasm, cortical granules are rare or occur in scattered clusters. By contrast, the GV-stage oocyte show in Figure 71a is a representative example of a more typical GV cytoplasm in which cortical granules occur at high density and mitochondria are both more numerous and uniformly distributed. Cortical granules can be visualized with fluorescent probes and their density and distribution determined by scanning laser confocal microscopy. Figure 71b is a confocal microscopic image through the approximate center of a GV-stage oocyte showing what is considered a normal density of cortical granules.

One of the earliest events in the preovulatory meiotic maturation of the mammalian oocyte is the rapid disappearance of the nucleolus followed shortly thereafter by the dissolution of the nuclear membrane. This stage of meiotic maturation is termed germinal vesicle breakdown (GVBD) and is preceded by an abrupt cessation of detectable transcription that is temporally associated with nucleolar dissolution. At the fine structural level, the termination of transcription is the result of the disappearance of the granular component of the nucleolus that is involved in the synthesis of ribosomal and transfer RNA. A well-developed granular component of the prominent oocyte nucleolus and a highly porous nuclear membrane are two characteristics of actively growing rather than fully grown oocytes. Interestingly, these two characteristics are common in GV-stage human oocytes that occur in fully grown follicles after COHS and ovulation induction (for IVF) (Figure 72a, b). Although such oocytes can spontaneously resume meiosis and mature to MII *in vitro*, if fertilized, embryo performance is frequently abnormal and ongoing pregnancies after IVF are very rare. Although the etiology of developmental incompetence is unknown, one possibility suggests that, in these instances, ovulation induction promotes cytoplasmic but not nuclear maturation. Temporal and spatial asynchronies in the expression of these fundamental developmental programs could have lethal downstream consequences that may not become apparent until the pre- and early postimplantation stages of embryogenesis.

Similar to fine structural descriptions of oocyte mitochondria in other mammals[53], mitochondria in fully grown human oocytes are small ($\leq 0.4\,\mu m$), ellipsoidal/spheroidal structures whose few cristae rarely penetrate a dense inner matrix (Figure 71c). Despite a TEM appearance that is consistent with an under- or undeveloped state, these mitochondria are metabolically active and are a major, if not primary source of energy (i.e. ATP) for the oocyte and early

preimplantation-stage embryo[54,55]. Determinations of the number of mitochondria/oocyte that have used morphometric algorithms to count mitochondria in representative thin sections, suggest that the normal human MII oocyte may contain about 150 000 organelles[55]. Recent quantitative analyses of the mitochondrial DNA (mtDNA) content of MII human oocytes indicate copy numbers ranging from 20 000 to nearly 1 000 000[55]. If each mitochondrion contains a single mtDNA molecule, as is currently assumed, the mitochondrial complement of oocytes within the same cohort could differ by well over an order of magnitude! This possibility needs to be confirmed by morphometric analysis of human oocytes that, in the living state, appear to have very different cytoplasmic densities, as measured by the intensity of mitochondrial staining with non-toxic, organelle-specific (fluorescent) probes[56].

Mitochondria are maternally inherited organelles that are not thought to undergo duplication until after implantation. Therefore, as the embryo develops through the preimplantation stages, mitochondrial numbers/cell would be expected to be halved with each cell division, assuming their segregation between daughter cells is uniform. It might be suspected that, if a comparatively low mitochondrial complement size exists at fertilization, negative consequences for embryo competence could occur if their number is insufficient to provide levels of ATP required for morphogenetic processes (e.g. cavitation) and biosynthetic activities[56]. Indeed, a reduced mitochondrial complement in human oocytes has been a suggested cause of maturational arrest during the preovulatory stages and may be a contributing factor to some fertilization and early embryonic failures in clinical IVF[57].

The apparent differences in mitochondrial density observed by TEM between human GV-stage oocytes may be developmentally significant if those with seemingly low numbers have a corresponding reduced competence for maturation, fertilization or normal embryogenesis. At present, selected TEM images of human oocytes, such as those shown here or in other fine structural studies[58], cannot provide meaningful quantitative information concerning the number of mitochondria present in the sectioned oocyte. Consequently, quantitative determinations of mitochondria and what could be considered a complement size consistent with normal competence await a systematic morphometric (TEM) analysis of representative mature (MII) and immature (GV) oocytes obtained from different cohorts of fully grown follicles. If a subnormal mitochondrial complement is reflected by low mtDNA copy numbers and confirmed to be a cause of maturational or embryonic developmental incompetence, it will become relevant to ask whether the occurrence of unusually high mtDNA copy numbers has developmental consequences as well. Perhaps the most interesting question to be addressed by those currently engaged in the study of mitochondria and early human development is a mechanistic one, namely, how can such apparently huge differences in mitochondrial and mtDNA numbers arise during oogenesis?

The injection of a single dose of human chorionic gonadotropin (hCG) has long been used to induce ovulation in cycles of COHS where its administration at high levels is designed to mimic the natural LH surge. For the oocyte, the principal aim of ovulation induction is to affect the simultaneous resumption of maturation in GV-stage oocytes contained within multiple follicles such that when aspirated shortly before ovulation is anticipated (typically some 38–40 hours post-hCG), most will have achieved meiotic maturity (i.e. MII) and completed cytoplasmic maturation. In the latter instance, the issue of whether all oocytes have completed maturation at retrieval is controversial, but it is generally assumed that both meiotic and cytoplasmic maturation will be largely completed if oocytes are cultured for a few hours prior to insemination. For many women undergoing infertility treatment by COHS and IVF, only a small fraction of oocytes retrieved after ovulation induction remains at the GV stage. For others, however, the fraction of immature oocytes can be sizeable and, as a result, adversely affect the probability of a successful outcome owing to the reduced number of oocytes available for fertilization. TEM examination of residual immature oocytes can be particularly useful in understanding the origins of developmentally lethal cytoplasmic defects that often affect their meiotically mature (MII) siblings[59,60]. In this respect, such information can be clearly important in understanding certain etiologies of infertility if defects that arise during oogenesis can be distinguished from those that develop because of follicular stimulation or after ovulation induction. For example, extensive vesiculation is a common defect observed in MII-stage oocytes aspirated from fully grown follicles[59,60]. The occurrence of a similar phenotype in GV-stage oocytes derived from the same cohort(s) suggests

that vesiculation of this type may not preclude nuclear maturation, i.e. the defect detected at MII may have originated at the GV stage. However, the structural characteristics of these vacuoles in both MII- and GV-stage human oocytes (Figure 73) suggest that they are distended cisternae of the SER. Perturbation of SER function could have adverse, if not toxic downstream consequences for embryogenesis, owing to the participation of the SER in the regulation of intracellular free calcium levels (see below). At present, it is assumed that this defect is the result of an atypical response of the oocyte cytoplasm to COHS rather than an inherent defect that developed during earlier stages of oogenesis.

Figure 73 illustrates another common aspect of cellular organization in human GV-stage oocytes that failed to mature after ovulation induction, namely, the occurrence of multiple defects. In this instance, in addition to cytoplasmic vacuoles, no nucleolus is detected (confirmed by serial section analysis) and a good portion of the zona pellucida is disorganized or malformed such that it seems to penetrate the ooplasm deeply at several locations. The absence of a nucleolus suggests that nuclear maturation may have been initiated after hCG administration, but arrested prior to GVBD. Although speculative at present, it is an intriguing possibility that abnormal calcium signaling associated with a perturbed SER network could block the progression of nuclear maturation (i.e. meiosis) by failing to promote the dissolution of the germinal vesicle membrane. One of the regions of the cortical ooplasm penetrated by this aberrant zona pellucida is shown at high magnification in Figure 74. TEM analysis shows apparently normal coronal cells whose transzonal processes appear intact and continuous as they course through an unusually thickened and elongated invagination of the zona pellucida and contact the oolemma. While the etiology of this phenotype remains to be determined, it seems unlikely to be caused by unusual intrafollicular physical conditions that arise during COHS or following the administration of an ovulatory dose of hCG. The finding that the length of the transzonal processes, from coronal cell origin to oolemmal termination, is significantly longer in this region than where the thickness and organization of the zona pellucida is normal, strongly suggests that the defect arises during the early stages of the biogenesis of the zona pellucida and is therefore a pre-existing structural defect. However, the localization of this defect to a portion of the zona pellucida and corresponding ooplasm raises questions about the normality of communication between germ and somatic cells by means of the corresponding transzonal processes. Compromised or abnormal communication could be one explanation for the failure of these oocytes to mature *in vivo*.

Studies of the fertilization process in model systems such as the mouse show that the ability of sperm to attach to the oolemma and enter the ooplasm are aspects of cytoplasmic maturation that develop during the terminal stages of the preovulatory period. However, this does not seem to be the case for the human because a very significant fraction of GV-stage oocytes aspirated from fully grown follicles (Figure 75a) have been shown to be penetrated by spermatozoa after insemination *in vitro*[61]. In these instances, nuclear immaturity could not be readily determined prior to insemination owing to the enclosure of the oocyte by a dense corona radiata and cumulus oophorus layer. This surprising phenomenon of sperm penetration in GV-stage human oocytes is especially evident after staining with DNA-specific fluorescent probes with imaging of the oocyte in 1–5-µm serial sections by means of scanning laser confocal microscopy, such as those shown in Figure 75b–d.

During the normal course of preovulatory nuclear maturation, nucleolar dissolution is followed by the initiation of chromatin condensation into chromosomes at discrete foci along the circumference of the inner nuclear membrane. Shortly after chromatin condensation begins, the dissolution of the nuclear membrane or 'germinal vesicle breakdown' occurs. Chromatin condensation continues in the absence of an intact nuclear envelope and ends with the formation of discrete bivalent chromosomes. Because the pattern of DNA condensation follows the general topology of the former spherical nucleus, the bivalent chromosomes are distributed in a comparatively radial fashion in the region formerly occupied by the germinal vesicle. As a result of the largely circumferential arrangement of chromosomes, in conventional cytogenetic preparations in which chromosomes are fixed onto a slide, this phase of nuclear maturation has been traditionally known as the circular bivalent stage (CBV). For human oocytes, the CBV stage is often detected in those oocytes that spontaneously resume meiosis *in vitro* after recovery at the GV stage from fully grown follicles. The three examples shown in Figure 75b–d are oocytes that had been penetrated by a single spermatozoon (arrows) at the GV stage and were analyzed by scanning laser confocal microscopy after staining with DNA-specific fluorescence molecules shortly after GVBD. An organized distribution of bivalent chromosomes at the CBV stage is also necessary for the proper attachment of kinetochore microtubules to the bivalent chromosomes that leads to normal equatorial alignment of the chromosomes on the metaphase I meiotic spindle. Segregation of the bivalents into monovalent chromosomes signals the completion of meiosis I with one set of chromosomes remaining in the oocyte and the other discharged in a small nucleoplast, the first polar body. Nuclear maturation progresses to metaphase II (MII) at which stage it is arrested and not reinitiated unless the oocyte is activated by sperm penetration or experimental manipulations. A large proportion of numerical chromosomal disorders (aneuploidy) observed in early human embryos results from segregation errors (premature chromatid separation, anaphase lag, non-disjunction) that arise during preovulatory nuclear maturation[3,28]. For clinical purposes, the most important element with respect to infertility treatments that use IVF is the occurrence of chromosomally normal MII oocytes in follicular aspirates obtained after COHS and ovulation induction.

THE METAPHASE II STAGE OF THE OOCYTE

The frequency with which immature oocytes occur in cycles of COHS and ovulation induction is specific for the patient and cycle (cohort). For IVF, human oocytes suitable for insemination are those that have responded to ovulation induction and reinitiated maturation *in vivo* and, at retrieval, have completed nuclear maturation to MII; and cytoplasmic maturation, as demonstrated by the acquisition of maximum ability to block polyspermic penetration and competence to decondense sperm DNA and promote male and female pronuclear evolution. As discussed in Chapter 4, defects in each of these activities can occur within cohorts of oocytes subjected to IVF. Typically, the status of nuclear maturation is difficult to determine after follicular aspiration, because the oocyte is normally obscured by coronal and cumulus cells (Figure 76a). In conventional IVF, confirmation of meiotic status usually occurs many hours after insemination, when the surrounding granulosa cells are mechanically removed to confirm fertilization by virtue of the presence of two pronuclei. Several techniques that rely on the partial displacement of cumulus cells have been used with variable efficacy to stage meiosis in order to select only MII oocytes for insemination. In one method, passage of the oocyte/cumulus complex through a micropipet whose bore is slightly larger than the oocyte can frequently displace cumulus cells sufficiently so that direct visualization of the oocyte is possible (Figure 76b). If the cumulus oophorus is well expanded and relatively translucent, this procedure permits visualization of the first polar body and can often detect certain cytoplasmic defects associated with developmental incompetence. In contrast, intracytoplasmic sperm injection (ICSI) requires that these somatic cells be removed by a combination of enzymatic (hyaluronidase) and physical treatments in order directly to observe the meiotic status (i.e. MII) of the oocyte prior to its insemination by the mechanical placement of a spermatozoon within the ooplasm with a micropipet. Figure 76c shows a normal-appearing MII oocyte as observed by low-resolution light microscopy approximately 15 minutes after insemination by conventional IVF. A distinct and intact first polar body, a cytoplasm of relatively uniform texture, and an actively motile spermatozoon in the process of progressing through the zona pellucida are characteristics favorable for normal fertilization.

Clinical experience from over 25 years of IVF demonstrates that the unique developmental potential of the embryo is largely established in the oocyte during preovulatory maturation. This is certainly the case for structural and numerical chromosomal disorders, whose detection prior to ICSI requires fluorescent *in situ* hybridization (FISH) analysis of the chromosomal complement of the first polar body[15,62]. Considerable research efforts have been applied to the identification of morphological characteristics of MII oocytes that have high predictive value with respect to embryo competence. Indeed, morphological assessments of MII oocytes are preferred in most clinical settings because they are non-invasive. However, their efficacy requires that they accurately reflect normal and abnormal characteristics that can be clearly supported by clinical outcomes. With regard to efficacy, results from tens of thousands of oocyte inspections present a mixed picture. MII oocytes whose competence can be established by outcome after embryo transfer show a

range of cytoplasmic phenotypes and, because morphological assessments are subjective or operator-dependent, their utility in clinical IVF is often controversial. Subtle differences in cytoplasmic appearance (e.g. texture, density) that may be considered problematic for development by one operator may fall within the normal range for another. At present, there is no ideal morphology for MII human oocytes that can be unambiguously correlated with chromosomal normality (euploidy), developmental competence after fertilization, and the ability of the embryo to develop progressively through gestation to birth. While the derivation of clinically relevant associations between subtle aspects of oocyte morphology detected prior to fertilization and outcome after embryo transfer is an ongoing research process, oocyte selection schemes for infertility treatment need to be objective and, if morphologically based, understood in the context of corresponding molecular or biochemical defects that may be expressed morphologically.

In contrast, there are certain structural and organization defects common to MII human oocytes obtained by COHS for IVF that are clearly associated with reduced competence[3,19,20,28,59,60]. For example, an area of focal cytoplasmic disorganization (asterisk, Figure 77a, b) results from abnormal aggregations or clustering of organelles such as mitochondria and distended SER cisternae. After DNA staining of affected oocytes, fluorescence microscopic analysis frequently shows disruption of the meiotic spindle or chromosomal scattering, or both (Figure 77b). Embryos resulting from such oocytes often arrest development *in vitro* or show very high frequencies of post-implantation loss that are currently thought to be associated with lethal chromosomal defects. In contrast, a normal MII human oocyte is largely considered to have a cytoplasm of uniform texture and a discrete and intact first polar body (Figure 77c) that overlies a MII spindle in the subjacent cortical ooplasm (Figure 77d). As noted above, however, this 'ideal' appearance is not synonymous with euploidy and, in practice, such oocytes often contain numerical chromosomal defects that arose during preovulatory meiotic maturation[62].

Vacuolation is another potentially lethal phenotype commonly observed in MII oocytes after cycles of COHS (Figure 78a, b). In particular, the occurrence of one or two large fluid-filled vacuoles can be developmentally lethal if they persist during the first cell division, owing to the distortion of the plane of cleavage that produces uneven blastomeres and adversely effects the normality of chromosomal and organelle segregation. An aberrant endocytotic mechanism in which fluid uptake from the perivitelline space is rapid and uncontrolled has been a suggested etiology of this defect, although time-lapse studies indicate that smaller vacuoles often coalesce to form one or more larger inclusions. An extreme example of this defect observed by TEM is shown in Figure 78c and at higher magnification in Figure 78d. These images seem to include the original site of dysfunction (indicated by an asterisk in Figure 78c) that led to the enormous accumulation of fluid and subsequent severe cytoplasmic distortion of this MII oocyte. The finding that oocytes with severe vacuolation are often at MII when retrieved from fully grown antral follicles suggests that the defect arises during the later stages of preovulatory maturation and may have an etiology related to the same type of zona defect described above for fully grown GV-stage oocytes (see Figure 73).

The occurrence of one or more disc-like structures readily identifiable by light microscopy by virtue of their shape and relative translucency is a third common cytoplasmic phenotype associated with reduced competence for MII human oocytes obtained for IVF after COHS (asterisk, Figure 79). Fine structural studies demonstrate that these inclusions are dense accumulations of SER cisternae (Figure 79b) that are often enclosed by a circumferential layer of mitochondria (Figure 79c)[3,59]. Developmental lethality has been indicated by poor performance in vitro and high frequencies of postimplantation demise after embryo transfer[3]. While the etiology of this defect remains to be determined, developmental dysfunction may be associated with abnormalities in critical developmental events that are regulated by the SER, including transient and stage-specific changes in focal levels of intracellular free calcium[55]. The ability of SER cisternae to sequester and release calcium is currently thought to be one of the principal mechanisms by which intracellular levels of this cation are regulated in the oocyte and early embryo[55,63]. Calcium is involved in critical and diverse cellular processes such as the regulation of the cell cycle, spindle formation and function, levels of mitochondrial ATP production and perhaps the expression of certain signal transduction pathways that mediate differential genomic transcription[55,64]. It is unknown whether SER function and calcium homeostasis are perturbed in human oocytes and

newly fertilized eggs exhibiting this cytoplasmic phenotype. However, a recent study of affected oocytes confirmed previous findings that the discs are atypical assemblages of SER, and their occurrence prior to IVF results in embryos that undergo early demise in vitro at very high frequency and, if developmentally progressive during culture, fail to implant after uterine transfer[65]. The single birth that resulted from an affected oocyte in this study was an infant with a genomic imprinting disorder that was suggested to be associated with abnormal SER function, possibly related to the regulation of cytoplasmic free calcium. This disturbing finding strongly dictates against their insemination in infertility treatment that uses IVF. While affected oocytes can be fertilized by means of ICSI, abnormalities in calcium regulation at the earliest stages of embryogenesis have been shown in experimental systems to have lethal downstream consequences that become evident during the postimplantation stages of organogenesis[66]. The importance of TEM analysis is clearly validated in the case of this SER defect because of its potential association with the ability of the oocyte and early preimplantation-stage embryo to regulate intracellular calcium.

The search for definitive morphological markers of human oocyte competence in general, and specific characteristics that can be correlated with putative genetic or other developmentally significant defects in particular, has been an ongoing effort in clinical IVF for over 25 years. Today, this research has become especially relevant in countries where the number of oocytes that can be inseminated or embryos transferred is legally stipulated, and the use of genetic analysis or cryopreservation in infertility treatment prohibited. While TEM has been especially effective in understanding the subcellular basis of overt oocyte defects, it also enables subtle differences in cytoplasmic organization and structure to be identified between oocytes that appear grossly normal and morphologically equivalent at the light microscopic level. The important issues are whether these differences are developmentally significant and, if so, whether they can be detected by noninvasive methods. For example, the colorized electron micrographs shown in Figures 80 and 81 demonstrate the analytical power of TEM when applied to the study of MII human oocytes that appeared normal by light microscopy. Differential colorization allows specific cellular components to be viewed in the context of their spatial distribution and interrelationships within the cytoplasm. Subcellular features of human oocytes largely assumed to be consistent with developmental competence include the following: (1) a relatively uniform distribution of mitochondria within a cytoplasm free of disorganization or structural anomalies; (2) a distinct complement of cortical granules (CG) distributed throughout the circumference of subplasmalemmal cytoplasm; and (3) a well-formed, barrel-shaped MII spindle located beneath the first polar body in which (4) chromosomes are equatorially aligned on the spindle microtubules. The importance of TEM in the ongoing analysis of cytoplasmic factors that may contribute to developmental competence is well illustrated in these two representative micrographs that, as noted above, are derived from normal-appearing MII oocytes. What they reveal, however, are structural differences in the organization and symmetry of the MII spindle, differences in the concentration and distribution of cortical granules, and apparent numerical and spatial differences associated with the SER. Structural differences in the organization of the meiotic metaphase spindle can lead to chromosomal malsegregation (non-disjunction and anaphase lag) at metaphase I or II that will result in embryos with numerical chromosomal disorders (aneuploidy). The colorized images of MII spindles seen in Figures 80 and 81, and at higher magnification in Figure 82c, d, represent two common phenotypes detected at the fine structural level in MII human oocytes obtained in IVF treatment cycles.

TEM is not the preferred method of analysis for studying meiotic spindle organization and structure when large numbers of human oocytes are involved. Research into the relationship between spindle abnormalities and certain etiologies of infertility, including advanced maternal age[29,67,68], have used fluorescence microscopy to visualize the spindle and associated chromosomes after fixation and staining with molecular probes specific for each component. Two representative examples of meiotic spindles in grossly normal-appearing MII-stage human oocytes stained with anti-tubulin antibodies (red fluorescence, microtubules) and DNA-specific probes (chromosomes, blue fluorescence) and imaged by scanning laser confocal microscopy are shown in Figure 82a, b. Differences in chromosomal location and alignment, the organization and distribution of spindle fibers (i.e. microtubules), and the overall shape, symmetry and structure of the spindle, could lead to a classification of normal and abnormal, respectively.

Interpretations of spindle normality or abnormality by fluorescence microscopy are validated at the subcellular level by the detection of similar structural and organizational characteristics associated with normal (Figure 82c) or abnormal designations (Figure 82d). The clinical importance of this validation in infertility treatments that require IVF is related to the current use of polarized optics to visualize spindles in living oocytes by virtue of the birefringent properties of organized spindle microtubules[69,70]. In some instances, computerized enhancement and processing of polarized images can clearly identify abnormal spindles similar in structure and organization to those described above. With validation by TEM and conventional fluorescence microscopy, imaging spindles in human MII oocytes with computer-enhanced polarizing optics may permit the classification of oocytes into groups that have high or low aneuploidy potential prior to insemination.

The differential morphology of the human oocyte MII spindle is one of the best examples to date of how fine structural aspects of normality and abnormality have the potential to be recognized by novel non-invasive light microscopic methods that can then be applied in infertility treatment. TEM analysis of mature human oocytes also demonstrates differences in other cellular components that have been suggested to be of developmental significance, most notably, mitochondria and the SER. The organization and distribution of the SER may be a particularly critical determinant of competence for the oocyte and the preimplantation-stage embryo, because of its role in the regulation of intracellular free calcium. The SER occurs in the human MII-stage oocyte as discrete spherical assemblages of cisternae (colored orange in Figures 80 and 81) that in normal oocytes are always in proximity to or surrounded by mitochondria (colored blue in these figures). It has been proposed that this pattern of SER/mitochondrial association forms complexes that regulate both local levels of free calcium and mitochondrial ATP production[55,64]. Although speculative at present, it is an intriguing notion that SER/mitochondrial complexes located in the subplasmalemmal cytoplasm, such as the one shown in Figure 83a, may be responsive to transmembrane ionic and electrical fluxes that occur when a sperm attaches to the oolemma and, if responsive, could mediate developmentally critical calcium-dependent signal transduction pathways during the earliest stages of the fertilization process[71,72]. In the mouse oocyte, calcium release and sequestration involving the SER have been shown to up- or downregulate levels of oxidative phosphorylation and ATP production by mitochondria in proximity to these elements[64]. A similar functional relationship has been proposed for SER/mitochondrial complexes in the mature human oocyte, including the participation of mitochondria in the regulation of calcium homeostasis by virtue of the ability of these metabolically active organelles to sequester and release calcium as well[55]. The mitochondrial/ SER complex shown in Figure 83b is located in the interior portion of the ooplasm and, owing to the association between these two types of organelles, could be envisaged to form a 'functional respiratory complex' in which levels of ATP production can be rapidly adjusted by changes in ambient calcium levels.

Intracytoplasmic regions (domains) with different ambient ATP concentrations have been detected in certain differentiated somatic cells and correlated with corresponding differences in mitochondrial density and activity[72]. These findings suggest that transient domains of high and low ATP may be involved in the local regulation of energy-dependent processes such as enzymatic and biosynthetic activities, morphodynamic movements and intracellular circulation. A similar situation may exist in the mammalian oocyte during the normal progression of preovulatory maturation that leads to the acquisition of developmental competence. Stage-specific changes in mitochondrial distribution, density and perhaps association with other calcium-regulating elements such as the SER may establish intracellular conditions in the oocyte consistent with local control of multiple cytoplasmic activities and developmentally relevant processes. If SER/mitochondrial complexes are involved in the regulation of local free calcium and ATP levels in the human oocyte, one possibility is that the normality of nuclear and cytoplasmic maturation during the preovulatory stages, and perhaps the establishment of competence for embryogenesis after fertilization, involve stage-related changes in the relative density and specific distribution of these complexes. As shown in Figures 80 and 81, colorization of the cytoplasm in a manner that accentuates these complexes can be very useful in this regard. In these instances, the TEM images were taken at the same approximate depth in two MII oocytes that appeared normal by light microscopy. It is immediately evident that, at this level, the complexes are largely restricted to the cortical cytoplasm in one

oocyte (Figure 80) and located in both cortical and interior regions in the other (Figure 81). However, extrapolations of differential complex distribution to the entire cytoplasm or interpretations concerning developmental significance cannot be made from a few thin sections, even if taken at comparable levels in two different oocytes. What this type of analysis does provide is new information about subcellular organization that can suggest more detailed studies are warranted. In the case of the SER/mitochondrial complexes, for example, one impression obtained from the colorized images shown at high magnification in Figures 83a, b is that SER cisternae may extend into the cytoplasm from the central tubular matrix surrounded by mitochondria. The extent to which, if any, SER/mitochondrial complexes are interconnected and thus potentially capable of coordinated activity would require the ability to follow the intracytoplasmic progression of individual cisternae. The unique role of TEM in this type of study is demonstrated by its ability to enable portions of the cytoplasm to be reconstructed in detail simply by compiling multiple colorized images taken from serial (consecutive) thin sections.

As a research tool for studying the cell biology of human oogenesis, the utility of colorizing specific elements in TEM images is demonstrated by the clarity with which subtle interactions between cells (see also Chapters 1 and 2) and subcellular components can be visualized. For developmental significance to be established, however, living oocytes will require analysis by non-invasive methods that are capable of detecting differences in cellular interactions and organelle distribution/organization that can be associated with developmental abnormalities and failure. In this regard, the availability of molecular probes that target specific organelles such as mitochondria and SER in living cells may have significant applications in the study of human oocyte and embryo competence. For example, Figure 83b shows a living human MII oocyte stained with a SER-specific probe and examined by scanning laser confocal fluorescence microscopy[55]. This image displays all of the detectable SER complexes in the ooplasm in a single, two-dimensional projection. Analysis of representative 5-μm optical sections that were combined to form Figure 83b confirms TEM findings with respect to the discrete nature and spherical organization of SER complexes, as well as their differential size and distribution within the human ooplasm. This type of analysis can detect oocyte- and cohort-specific differences in the distribution, relative number and size of SER complexes that are comparable to findings obtained from individual TEM images, such as those shown in Figures 80 and 81. As discussed above, the importance of understanding SER function in the early embryo is demonstrated by clinical outcomes with conventional IVF and ICSI that have correlated abnormalities in SER organization at fertilization with high frequencies of pre- and postimplantation demise and, possibly, with DNA imprinting defects.

TEM studies will continue to identify subtle differences in cytoplasmic organization that contribute to differential oocyte and early embryo developmental competence. While these are valuable in understanding the cell biological origins of competence in general, fine structural information of this type will have clinical use in IVF only if specific states of organelle and cytoplasmic organization in oocytes and embryos are shown to be (1) clearly associated with competence and (2) detectable by non-invasive light microscopic methods that can be readily introduced in the IVF laboratory. The development of non-toxic probes and novel non-invasive microscopic methods that can reveal subtle cytoplasmic differences between oocytes represent a new and necessary avenue of investigation in clinical IVF. As shown here, TEM images can provide the fine structural context of competence-related intercellular and subcellular processes, activities and interactions, such as those between somatic granulosa cells and the oocyte, or between organelle systems in the ooplasm, that are currently thought to be critical determinants of developmental competence. It is also clear that differences in the biochemical and physiological milieu within the follicle can promote normal oocyte developmental competence at the cytoplasmic and chromosomal levels. Failure of competence-promoting conditions to develop during follicular growth and preovulatory maturation may be a significant factor contributing to the normal reduction in fertility and fecundity observed in women of advanced reproductive age and may also be an important etiology of idiopathic (unexplained) infertility in younger women. This may also be an important factor in outcome with infertility treatments that involve COHS and IVF because, within the same cohort of mature oocytes, a significant fraction of fertilized eggs may have inherited subtle cytoplasmic or numerical chromosomal defects whose adverse, if not lethal, effects on development may not be evident until late in the preimplantation phase or result in early postimplantation demise. As described above, follicle-specific differences in perifollicular blood flow rates that appear to reflect corresponding differences in the degree of expansion or patency of the perifollicular capillary bed have been related to oocyte competence. While Doppler ultrasonography can distinguish between follicles with differential blood flow indices, the extent to which, if any, different biochemical and physiological conditions that exist within follicles are reflected at the fine structural level remains to be investigated. TEM is an indispensable tool in this regard. It is currently the most sensitive method available to resolve subtle aspects of cytoplasmic organization and structure that can provide new insights into the cell biology of the oocyte as it relates to the establishment of developmental competence.

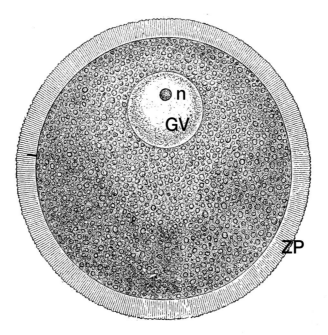

a

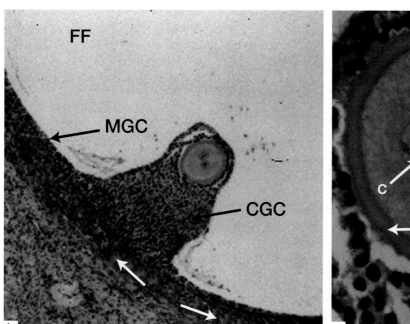

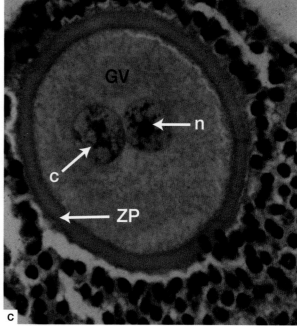

Figure 66 The structure of the immature human oocyte was accurately described in 19th century depictions as a large spherical cell (approximately 100 μm in diameter) containing a prominent nucleus that was termed the germinal vesicle (GV). Therefore, even today, the immature oocyte is said to be at the germinal vesicle stage. (a) Haeckel's original illustration of the human GV-stage oocyte in which a small spherical structure known as the nucleolus (n) is evident within the GV. As in all mammalian oocytes, the human oocyte is enclosed by an acellular 'shell' that, owing to its glass-like translucent appearance, was originally termed the zona pellucida (ZP) or clear zone. (b) and (c) are conventional light microscopic images of a human GV-stage oocyte in an antral follicle that was embedded in paraffin after fixation in formalin. The oocyte is positioned on a stalk-like mass of granulosa (follicle) cells termed the cumulus granulosa (CGC). The granulosa cells that line the wall of the follicle are termed mural granulosa cells (MGC) and are primarily responsible for steroid production, of which estrogen is the major product prior to ovulation. The follicular cavity or antrum is a cyst-like structure filled with fluid (follicular fluid, FF) that originates in part from serum transudation from perifollicular blood vessels (white arrows) and contains steroids secreted by the mural granulosa cells, and growth factors and other regulatory molecules that are both blood borne and locally produced by the cumulus granulosa cells. The oocyte shown in these figures is unusual as it is clearly binucleated rather than mononucleated, as is normal

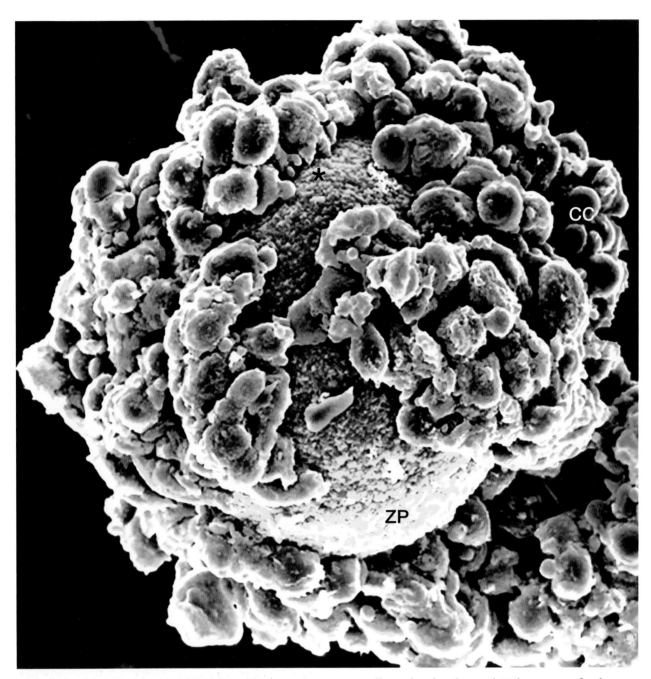

Figure 67 In a natural menstrual cycle, a single mature oocyte is usually ovulated each month. When *in vitro* fertilization (IVF) is used to treat infertility, current endocrine protocols exogenously manage the menstrual cycle with a variety of drugs and gonadotropins to effect the development of multiple follicles and their corresponding oocytes. This procedure is generally known as controlled ovarian hyperstimulation (COHS) and the occurrence of multiple and higher-order gestations (e.g. triplets) in certain infertility treatments is a direct consequence of the use of 'fertility drugs' that result in the production of multiple oocytes at ovulation (or retrieval for *in vitro* fertilization) and embryos after insemination. The SEM image of a human oocyte shown in this figure is characteristic of newly ovulated oocytes, regardless of whether nuclear and cytoplasmic maturation was completed. In this instance, most of the surrounding cumulus and coronal cells (CC) have been removed in order to visualize the surface of the zona pellucida (ZP). Typically, the oocyte could not be imaged directly owing to its encasement by the somatic follicle cells. The region indicated by an asterisk is shown at higher magnification in Figure 68

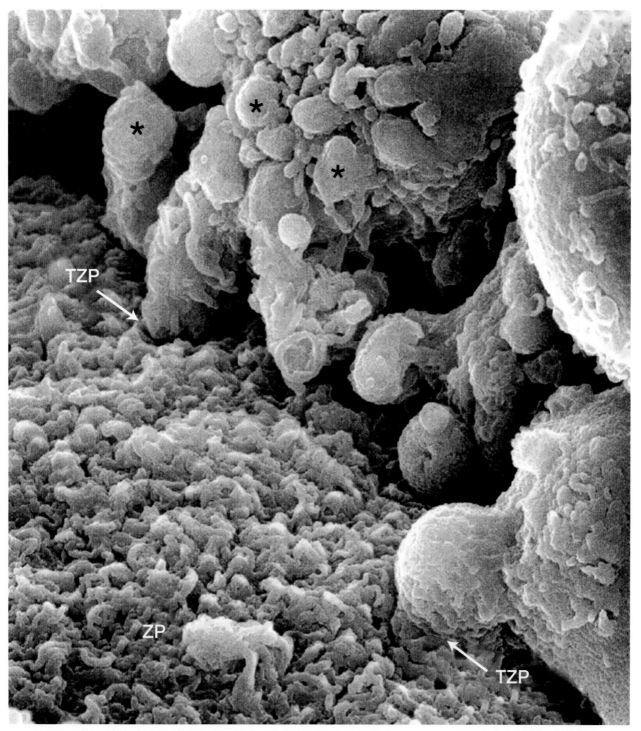

Figure 68 The virtue of imaging the surface of the oocyte at high magnification is that it provides a direct view of the acellular barrier through which the sperm must pass in order to fertilize the oocyte and also reveals features of the surrounding cells of the corona radiata that are probably related to biological activities that produce a normal oocyte. The coronal cells 'sit' on the surface of the zona pellucida (ZP) and, through elongated cytoplasmic extensions or processes that traverse this layer, directly contact the oocyte plasma membrane (the oolemma). The transzonal processes (TZP) are one of the primary means by which bidirectional communication between oocyte and follicle cells occurs and through which molecular information is exchanged. The surface architecture of the coronal cells also shows features that appear to be of a secretory nature. Most of these cells are decorated with protrusions commonly known as 'blebs' (asterisks) and are typical of cells known to export proteins and other molecules in small cytoplasmic compartments

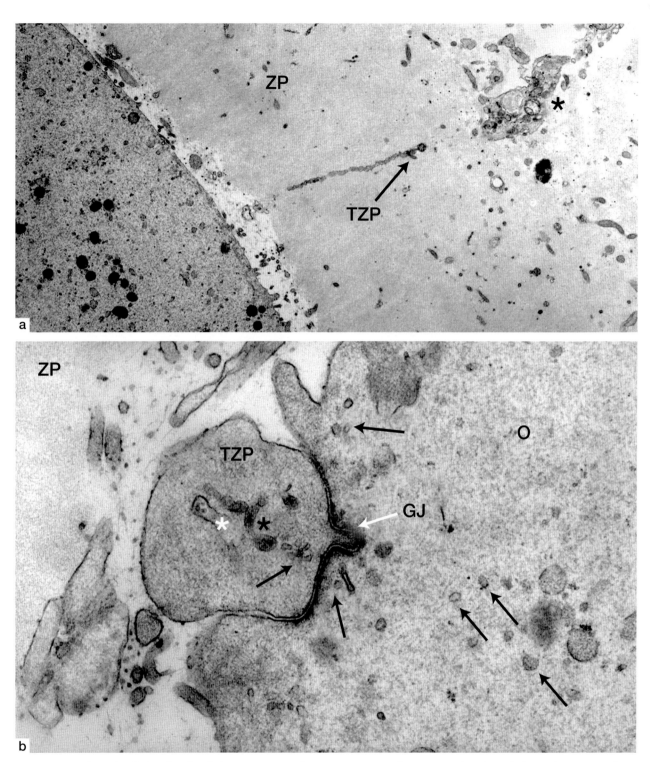

Figure 69 The subcellular details of the interactions between transzonal processes (TZP) and the oolemma are best revealed by TEM. (a) shows a portion of one of the numerous TZPs that traverse the zona pellucida (ZP), whose acellular structure is clearly evident in this electron micrograph. The cell body from which this transzonal process arises is indicated by an asterisk. (b) is a high-magnification view of the interaction between the oolemma and the 'foot' of a TZP. The presence of membrane-bound saccules (asterisks in TZP) and small vesicles (arrow in TZP) where their terminus or 'foot' contacts the oolemma is characteristic of the coronal cell processes. Direct communication between TZP and the oolemma involves gap junctions (GJ) whose structure permits bidirectional exchange of small molecules. The presence of a population of small vesicles in the oocyte (arrows in O) near the contact point of the TZP is of particular interest, as it suggests the possibility that vesicular traffic in both TZP and oocyte may also involve the exchange of molecular information through the processes by means of an endocytotic/exocytotic mechanism

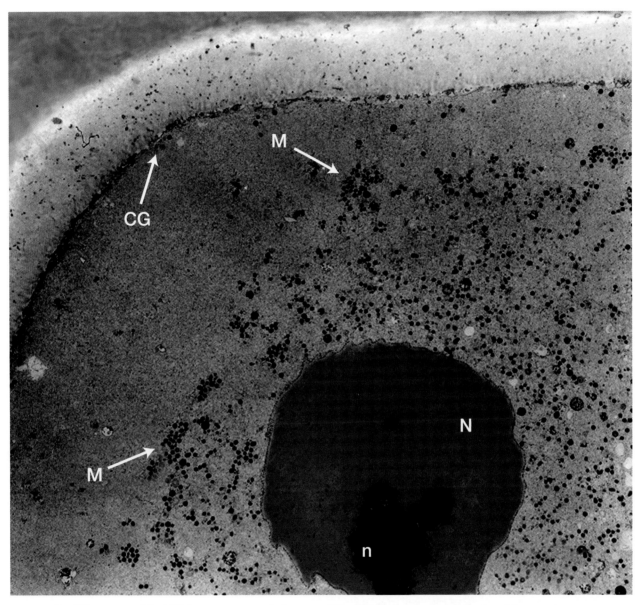

Figure 70 When viewed by TEM at comparatively low magnification, fully grown germinal vesicle-stage human oocytes appear to be relatively simple cells characterized by a prominent nucleus (N) that encloses an equally prominent nucleolus (n), and a cytoplasm in which small, spherical mitochondria (M), the organelles that provide energy (ATP) for the oocyte, are the most abundant component. Cortical granules (CG) are cytoplasmic elements whose contents are discharged (by exocytosis) into the space surrounding the oocyte (the perivitelline space) during the early stages of fertilization (termed the 'cortical reaction') and are largely responsible for the prevention of polyspermy, i.e. penetration by two or more spermatozoa. As evident from their name, cortical granules occur in the cortical cytoplasm and in normal oocytes form a continuous circumferential layer just beneath the oolemma

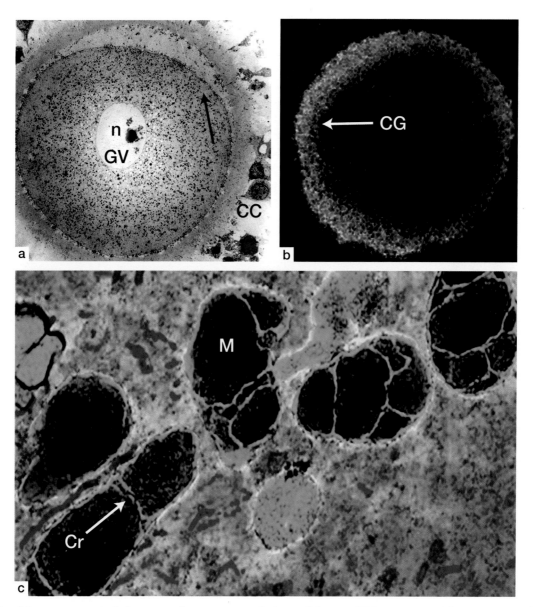

Figure 71   (a) is a comparatively low-magnification image of a 'typical' human GV-stage oocyte. The occurrence of cortical granules (CG) at high density is difficult to appreciate in a single thin section (arrow), but when living oocytes are stained with a cortical granule-specific fluorescent probe and imaged by scanning laser confocal microscopy (b), their high density is readily apparent even in a 2-μm optical section. Spontaneous exocytosis of cortical granules prior to insemination (premature 'cortical reaction') can induce hardening of the zona pellucida (premature 'zona reaction') and prevent the passage of a spermatozoon through this extracellular coat. The importance of these elements in the normal fertilization process is demonstrated by certain etiologies of infertility that have been attributed to premature cortical granule exocytosis. If premature cortical granule-induced zona hardening occurs in consecutive IVF attempts, it can be anticipated in a subsequent treatment cycle and often remedied by the mechanical insertion of a sperm using an invasive micromanipulation procedure termed ICSI (intracytoplasmic sperm injection). The numerous dark spheres shown in (a) are mitochondria, which are the most evident and abundant component of the oocyte cytoplasm, with numbers in normal human oocytes estimated to be in excess of 150 000. Although relatively active in ATP production, oocyte mitochondria (M) are rather small (approximately 0.4 μm in diameter) and undeveloped, as indicated in (c) by the presence of relatively few cristae (Cr) that penetrate a matrix of high electron density. Defects in mitochondrial function, or their occurrence at numbers significantly below normal (as may exist in the oocyte shown in Figure 70), have been associated with early human embryonic developmental arrest *in vitro* and have been suggested to contribute to early pregnancy loss after implantation

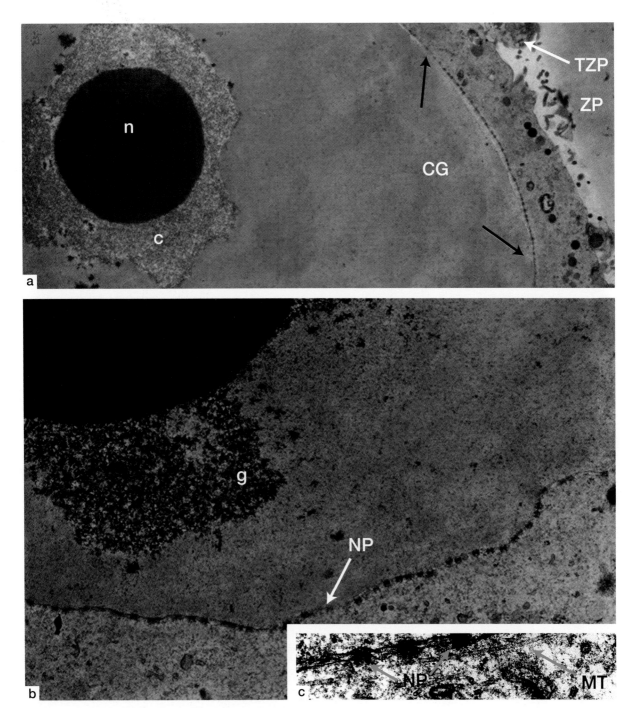

Figure 72 During the fetal stages of oogenesis, meiosis is arrested in GV-stage oocytes at prophase I. In natural menstrual cycles, meiosis I is resumed (reinitiated) after the LH surge and, in clinical IVF, this surge is mimicked by the administration of an ovulatory dose of human chorionic gonadotropin (hCG). For some older women undergoing ovulation induction for intrauterine insemination or IVF, this can mean that their oocytes have remained in meiotic arrest for over 40 years. The fine structural characteristics of the oocyte nucleus (the germinal vesicle) at the time of hCG administration are of particular interest as they can differ significantly between oocytes. For example, the occurrence of a granular component (g, b) suggests that RNA synthesis may be occurring, while in other oocytes, this component is absent or obscured by a pronounced halo of chromatin (c, a). The nuclear membrane of the GV-stage human oocyte can be a highly porous structure (NP, b) whose organization would seem to be one that promotes extensive molecular exchange between the cytoplasm and nucleoplasm. The high density of nuclear pores is clearly evident at higher magnification (NP, c) as are arrays of microtubules (MT) that occur throughout the circumference of the human germinal vesicle. Although the role(s) of these microtubules in the immature human oocyte is unknown, one possibility is that they provide a certain level of focal structure that may influence bidirectional molecular traffic between nucleus and cytoplasm. A circumferential layer of cortical granuals (CG, arrows) occurs beneath the oocyte plasma membrane

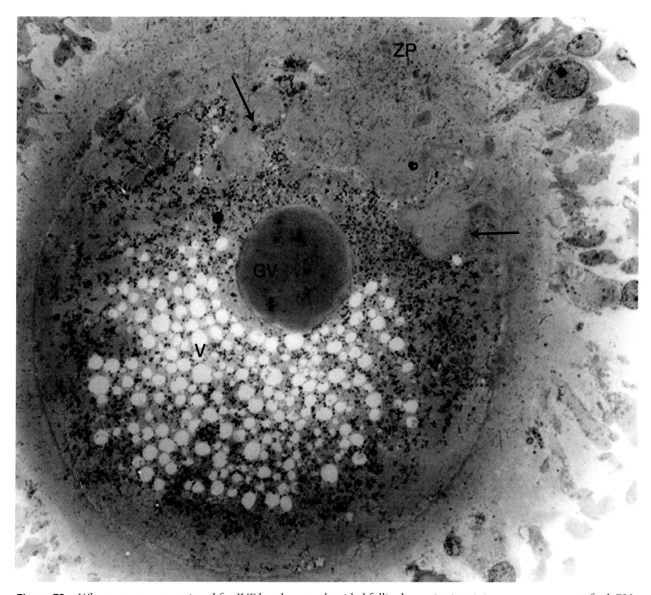

Figure 73 When oocytes are retrieved for IVF by ultrasound-guided follicular aspiration, it is not uncommon to find GV-stage oocytes some 36 hours after the administration of an ovulatory dose of hCG. Presumably, the oocyte or its surrounding coronal cells, or both, were unresponsive to ovulation induction *in vivo*. However, oocytes retrieved at the GV stage will often spontaneously resume meiosis *in vitro*. While the developmental competence of these 'in vitro matured' oocytes is questionable, what is unquestionable is that viability is compromised in GV oocytes that show the types of defects indicated in this figure. Here, the cytoplasm contains vacuoles (V) that are probably distended cisternae of the smooth-surfaced endoplasmic reticulum, and localized portions of the zona pellucida that have penetrated the ooplasm (arrows)

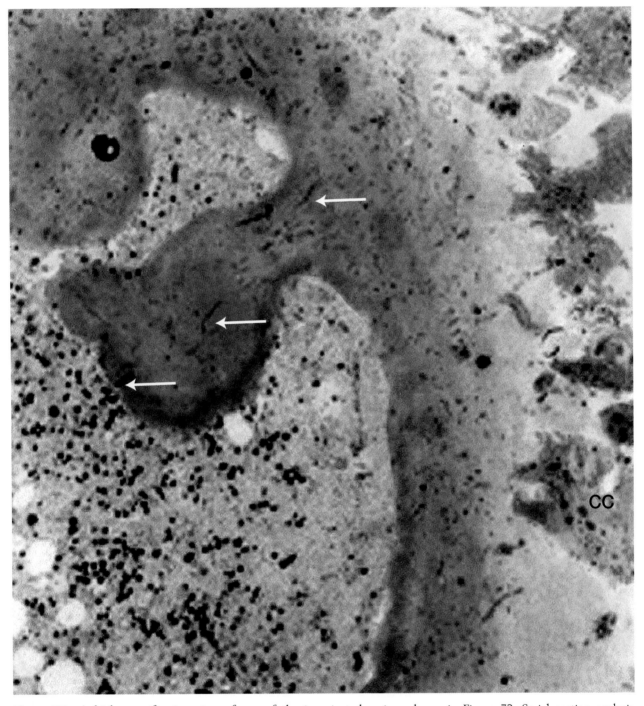

Figure 74 A high-magnification view of one of the invaginated regions shown in Figure 73. Serial section analysis demonstrates that the transzonal processes are unusually elongated (arrows) and are continuous from the follicle cell body to the oolemma in this region, suggesting that this unusual defect may have arisen when the zona was formed earlier in oogenesis. It is unknown whether communication between oocyte and coronal cells (CC) is normal or even functional in this disrupted region

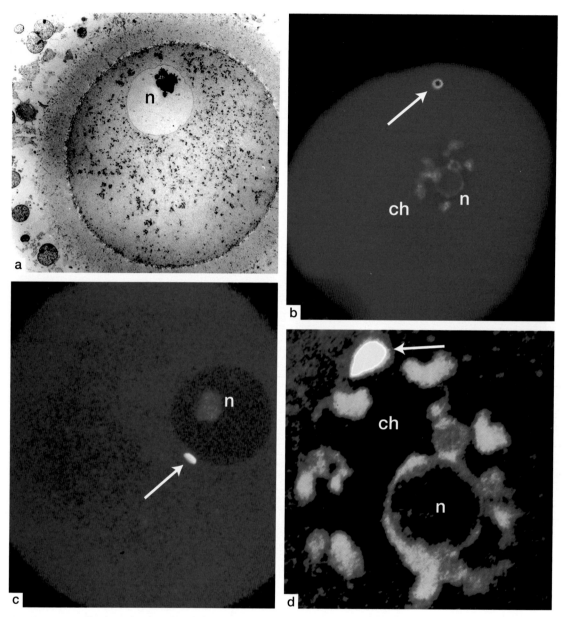

Figure 75 It is generally thought that the ability of a sperm to penetrate an oocyte is a fundamental aspect of cytoplasmic maturation that develops towards the end of the preovulatory phase, as nuclear maturation arrests at metaphase II and the follicle prepares for ovulation. (a) is a TEM image of a human GV-stage oocyte that failed to mature *in vivo* and was obtained by follicular aspiration 36 hours after the administration of an ovulatory dose of hCG. In the human, however, IVF results demonstrate that GV-stage oocytes such as these can be penetrated (b, c). In these instances, the sperm enters the cytoplasm and often migrates to come to rest on the nuclear membrane (c). The sperm nucleus remains in a condensed state in GV-stage oocytes that resume meiosis *in vitro*. For example, (b) shows a sperm nucleus (arrow) in an oocyte that was penetrated at the GV stage but which resumed meiosis *in vitro* and was imaged shortly after germinal vesicle breakdown (nuclear membrane dissolution) and the beginning of bivalent chromosomal condensation (ch). In these images, maternal and paternal DNA was stained with a specific fluorescent probe and resolved by scanning laser confocal microscopy. (d) shows another example of a sperm nucleus (arrow) that had progressed to the vicinity of the germinal vesicle and remained in a condensed state as meiotic maturation resumed *in vitro*

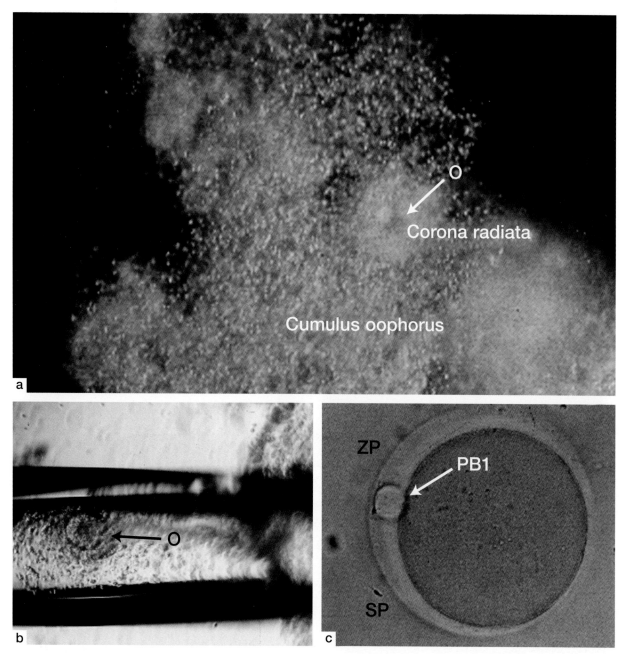

Figure 76 For IVF, oocytes are aspirated shortly before ovulation from fully grown human follicles that had been induced to ovulate with hCG. However, direct visualization of the newly recovered oocyte (O) is often difficult because it is generally surrounded by two layers of cells, the coronal radiation that resides on the surface of the zona pellucida and a significantly larger cumulus oophorus that surrounds the coronal layer (a). Several different techniques are used to facilitate inspection of the oocyte in the clinical IVF laboratory such as compression of the oocyte–cumulus complex in a glass pipette (b). If the cumulus oophorus is well expanded, inspection through the glass pipette can facilitate the direct visualization of the oocyte in order to determine whether a first polar body is present (an indication of meiotic maturity) and whether obvious defects in cytoplasmic organization exist. Alternatively, enzymatic and mechanical removal of coronal and cumulus cells prior to ICSI, or between 12 and 20 hours after insemination, when determinations of fertilization are made, will provide an unimpeded view of the oocyte (c). In general, a newly aspirated human oocyte is considered normal if the first polar body (PB1) is intact and the cytoplasm is relatively translucent and uniform in texture. The oocyte shown in (c) has been denuded of surrounding follicle cells prior to the addition of sperm and is shown within minutes following insemination. A single spermatozoon (SP) is already in the process of traversing the zona pellucida (ZP)

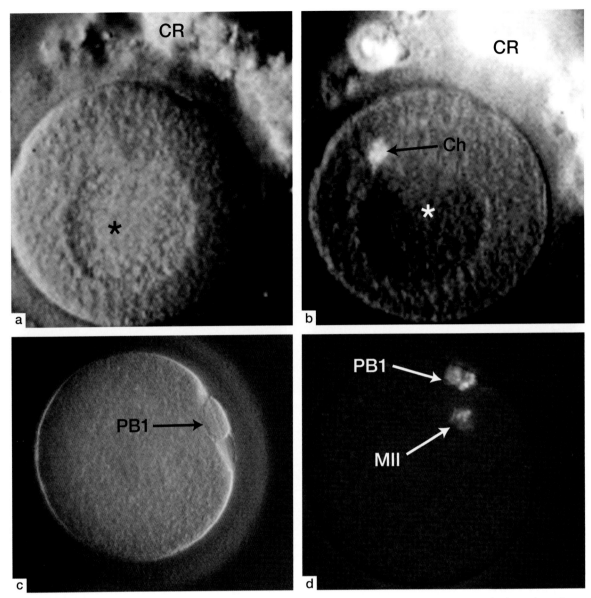

Figure 77 In clinical IVF, inspection of oocytes by light microscopy is the most common method used to determine whether cytoplasmic abnormalities or defects (termed cytoplasmic dysmorphisms) exist that would be expected to affect fertilization or embryonic development adverserly. Certain dysmorphisms observed at the time of insemination in meiotically mature human oocytes may be so evident that fertilization by conventional IVF or ICSI may not be warranted. An abnormal aggregation and clustering of organelles is one of the more frequent cytoplasmic dysmorphisms that affect human oocytes and in some instances can be so severe as to give the oocyte a 'bull's-eye' appearance (a, b). Usually, the metaphase II spindle (MII) is disorganized and the associated chromosomes (Ch) malaligned. In contrast, a presumably normal mature human oocyte (c) contains an intact polar body (PB1) and a cytoplasm free of evident disorganization or structural defects. The position of the MII spindle is also an important aspect of competence and is normally located in the cortical cytoplasm subjacent to the first polar body, as shown in (d). This image is the same as shown in (c) but was examined by fluorescence microscopy after staining with a DNA-specific probe (DNA fluoresces blue)

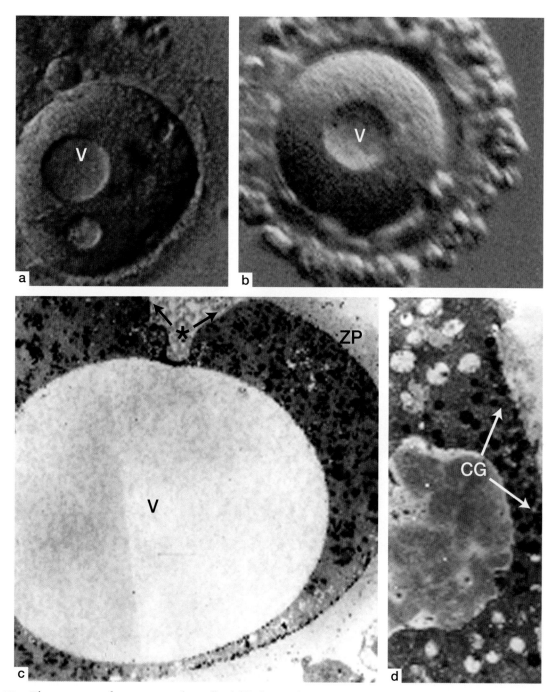

Figure 78   The presence of one or more large fluid-filled vacuoles (V) is another common human oocyte defect that can adversely influence developmental viability. This dysmorphism is clearly evident in the images shown here, where these inclusions occupy a significant proportion of the cytoplasm. In other instances, a few relatively small vacuoles may be developmentally benign and often can be detected in a single blastomere of an otherwise developmentally normal cleavage-stage embryo. The origin of this defect is unknown, although these vacuoles have been observed to develop rapidly in the oocyte and to undergo fusion. The transmission electron micrograph shown in (c) is an extreme example of vacuolation and, prior to fixation, several large vacuoles in this metaphase II oocyte were observed to coalesce into a single structure. It has been suggested that focal defects in the structure of the oocyte cortical cytoplasm may promote uncontrolled endocytosis of fluid from the perivitelline space and, in this oocyte, the region indicated by an asterisk in (c) is a likely site. At low magnification, it would also seem that a defect in the zona pellucida may be involved in the generation of these vacuoles. Although a zona defect cannot be precluded, this structure seems to be intact and normal at this location (arrows, c), as does the corresponding cytoplasm that, while remarkably thinned, does not appear degenerate and contains a dense cluster of cortical granules (d). Vacuolation is not as common as organelle clustering and the oocyte shown in (c) is a rare and extreme example of this dysmorphism. However, it is unknown how this abnormality arises or whether it is associated with certain intrafollicular conditions that develop during COHS stimulation for IVF

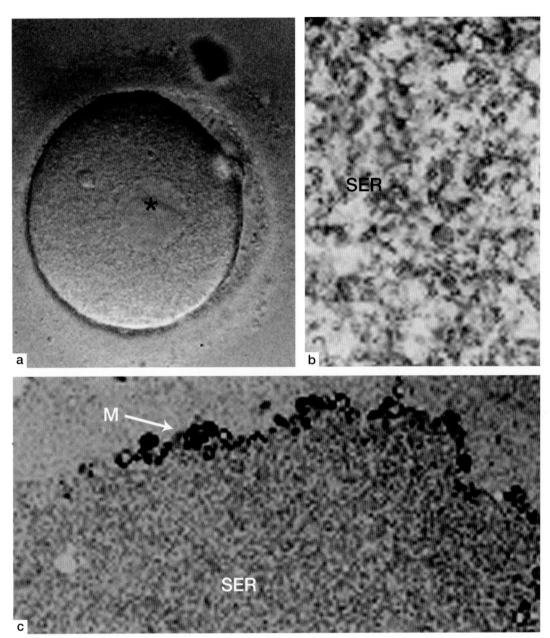

Figure 79 The presence of a relatively large and semitransparent disc-like structure (asterisk, a) is a third type of dysmorphism encountered in human oocytes obtained for IVF; its occurrence is invariably developmentally lethal. For some infertile women, virtually all of the mature oocytes aspirated from stimulated follicles are affected and it has been suggested that, for certain patients, this defect repeats on multiple IVF attempts. TEM demonstrates that this disc is an assemblage of elements of the smooth-surfaced endoplasmic reticulum (SER, b) that is surrounded by a layer of electron-dense mitochondria (M, c). While the origin of this defect is unknown, the role of the SER in calcium storage and release suggests that developmental lethality may be associated with an inability of the cytoplasm to regulate normal intracellular levels (maintain calcium homeostasis) of this cation which is involved in important cellular activities necessary for normal fertilization and embryogenesis, including regulation of the cell cycle and levels of mitochondrial ATP production

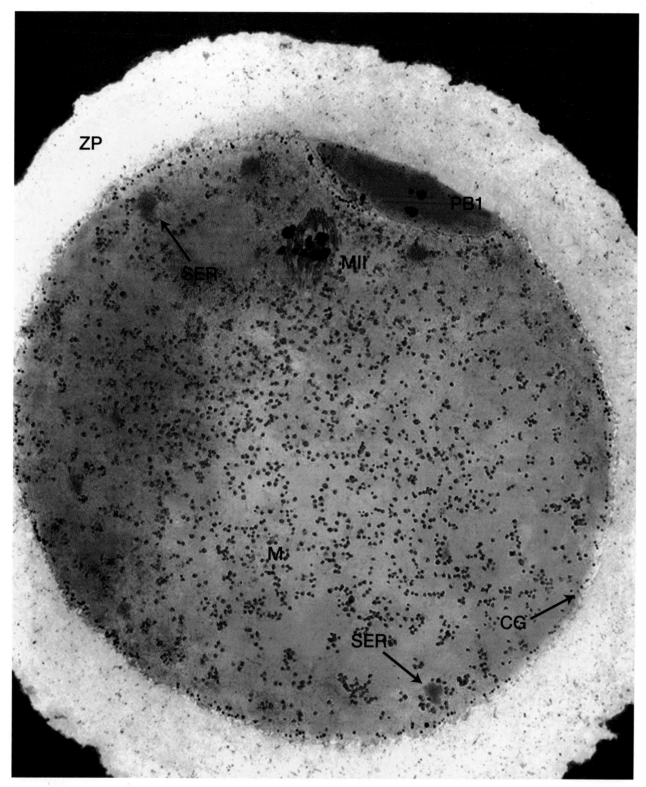

Figure 80 This relatively low-magnification TEM image of a mature metaphase II human oocyte depicts a typical pattern of cellular organization that is largely assumed to be associated with high developmental competence. Mitochondria are the most abundant organelles detected and typically occur in small clusters (M) throughout the cytoplasm. In this representative image, complexes of mitochondria and SER assemblages are observed just beneath the oolemma as well as in the cortical cytoplasm. A distinct, barrel-shaped meiotic spindle (MII) in which chromosomes are equatorially aligned is present in the cortical cytoplasm immediately beneath the first polar body (PB1). Cortical granules (CG) are distributed throughout the circumference of the subplasmalemmal cytoplasm

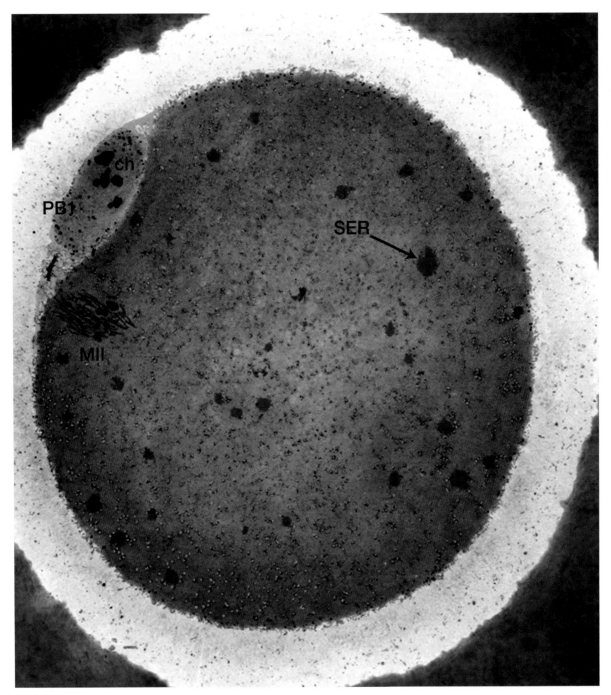

Figure 81 Similar to the electron micrograph shown in Figure 80, TEM imaging of this human MII stage oocyte at relatively low magnification shows organizational characteristics that are largely undetectable by conventional light microscopy. However, certain differences in the intracellular organization of this oocyte may be of developmental significance when compared to its sibling shown in Figure 80. Here, SER/mitochondrial complexes are present throughout the cytoplasm and the meiotic metaphase II (MII) spindle appears to be asymmetric with respect to the position of the chromosomes attached to the spindle microtubules. In serial sections, spindles of this type are elongated rather than barrel-shaped and often show abnormal patterns of chromosomal alignment that could be associated with aneuploidy or other chromosomal defects. The polar body is intact and contains a set of chromosomes that was eliminated at the end of the first meiotic division. When viewed at the light microscopic level, oocytes such as these appear normal with a cytoplasm of uniform texture. At the fine structural level, overall cytoplasmic normality is indicated by the absence of subtle structural defects or dysmorphisms associated with compromised developmental ability. It remains to be determined whether differences in the cytoplasmic distribution of SER/mitochondrial complexes between human oocytes are developmentally significant and, if so, whether their detection at the light microscopic level with organelle-specific fluorescent stains will be informative in this regard (see legend to Figure 83)

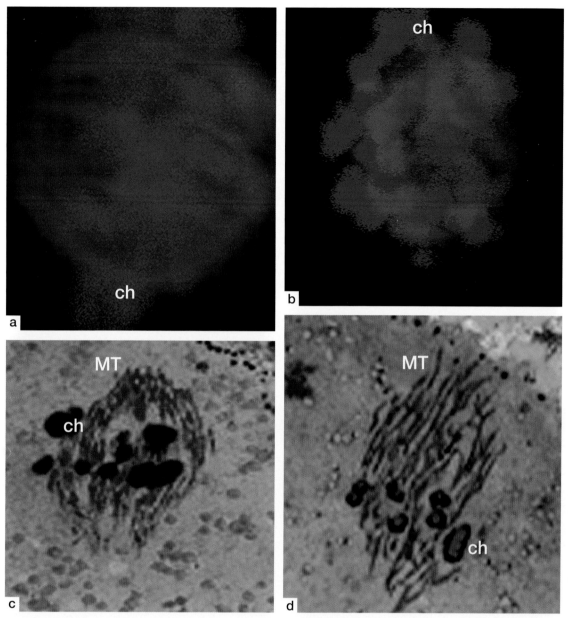

Figure 82 The structure and organization of the metaphase II spindle in the human oocyte is a critical determinant of the developmental normality of embryos, whether produced in natural menstrual cycles or in cycles involving assisted reproduction procedures such as IVF. There is considerable evidence that meiotic spindle disorders may exist at relatively high frequency in mature oocytes that appear normal at the light microscopic level, and that this frequency increases significantly with advancing reproductive age. (a) and (b) are fluorescent images of sibling oocytes staining with tubulin antibodies (red) and DNA-specific probes (blue) in order to resolve the structure and organization of the human MII spindle. These oocytes are representative examples of an apparently well-organized (a) and an obviously disorganized (b) MII spindle as imaged by scanning laser confocal fluorescence microscopy. In (b), chromosomes (ch) are not equatorially aligned and the spindle microtubules (MT) appear compact. (c) and (d) are high-magnification views of the spindles described for Figures 80 and 81, respectively, which show similar states of organization when viewed by TEM

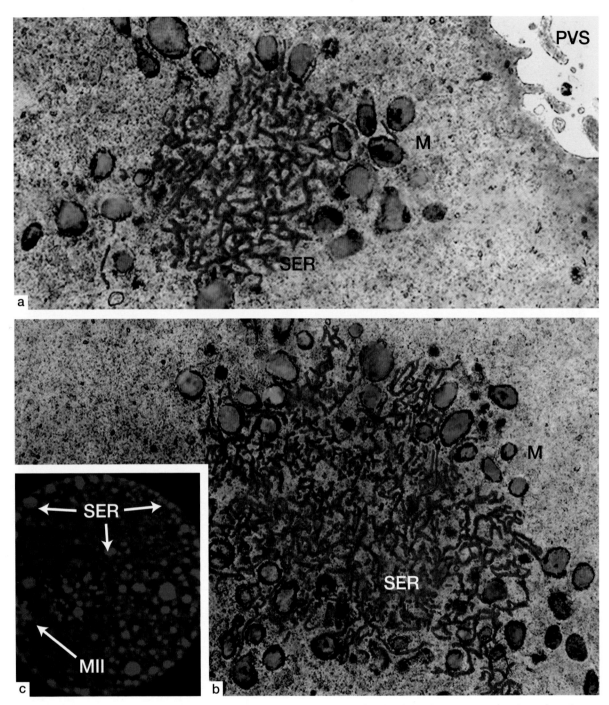

Figure 83 The smooth-surfaced endoplasmic reticulum (SER) plays a critical role in the oocyte and early embryo by virtue of its ability to regulate intracellular free calcium levels. In normal human oocytes, the SER is organized into discrete assemblages of elongated and interconnecting tubules that are surrounded by mitochondria (M). There is some indication from serial section reconstructions that discrete SER accumulations both in the cortical cytoplasm (a) and in the more interior regions of the cytoplasm (b) may be connected by means of extremely elongated tubules. If confirmed, this could suggest that spatially separated mitochondria/SER complexes may form discrete networks that respond to stimuli in a coordinated manner. For example, the association between mitochondria and SER suggests an arrangement that could be involved in the local intracellular regulation of mitochondrial ATP production, as calcium is a mediator of mitochondrial oxidative phosphorylation. It is unknown at present whether differences in the spatial distribution of SER/mitochondrial complexes, such as those shown in Figures 80 and 81, are of relevance with respect to developmental competence after fertilization. The SER can be visualized in living human oocytes cells with organelle-specific fluorescent probes, which confirms their spherical organization as seen by TEM and enables spatial differences in their distribution between oocytes to be identified (c). Such differences may be an important factor in the normality of the oocyte and if fertilized, the developmental competence of the oocyte. PVS, perivitelline space; MII, metaphase II chromosomes

4 The preimplantation stages of human embryogenesis

FERTILIZATION AND THE PRONUCLEAR STAGE

In natural conception and conventional IVF, sperm progress through the cumulus and coronal cells by a combination of (1) kinetic forces generated by a pattern of rapid tail motion that propels the sperm in a seemingly linear manner; and (2) the enzymatic activity of hyaluronidase, released from the acrosome during the so-called acrosome reaction. This enzyme catalyzes the breakdown of hyaluronic acid, the matrix substance in which cumulus cells are embedded, facilitating the progression of the sperm to the vicinity of the zona pellucida. Defects in sperm motility or the acrosome reaction can be important causes of male infertility. Insufficient ATP production from midpiece mitochondria may translate to sluggish motility and a significant reduction in the ability of spermatozoa to traverse the cumulus oophorus, even if hyaluronidase is discharged. In conventional IVF, where thousands or tens of thousands of motile spermatozoa are present at insemination, the vast majority never reaches the vicinity of the oocyte, as shown by the relatively small number of sperm found on the surface of the zona pellucida (Figure 84). Indeed, both real-time and time-lapse analyses of interactions between sperm and denuded human oocytes have long demonstrated that most sperm that contact the zona fail to attach or that the attachment is short-lived. These findings suggest that most of the human sperm prepared for *in vitro* fertilization are unable to form stable interactions with the zona pellucida or that the density of sperm attachment may be limited by the number of binding sites expressed at the zona surface. However, within and between cohorts, variation in the density of sperm–zona binding does occur and can be so extreme that, for some oocytes, nearly the entire surface of the zona is occupied by sperm. The stability of such intense binding is demonstrated by the persistence of accessory sperm through the cleavage stages, as shown at the 4-cell stage in Figure 85. Most often, embryos showing this sperm binding phenotype are polyspermic, as the intrinsic mechanisms the oocyte has developed to prevent multispermic penetration are simply overwhelmed by the numbers of highly motile sperm that have penetrated the zona pellucida and have attached to the oolemma at approximately the same time[73].

SEM findings show that the surface of the normal human zona pellucida displays a geometric structure composed of multiple ridge-like layers punctuated by numerous spaces or 'lacunae' of varying diameter (Figure 84). It is assumed that the structure of the zona observed in the fixed state, if not an artifact of dehydration, could indicate for the living oocyte an organization that may facilitate the attachment or passage of the fertilizing spermatozoon from the surface of the zona to the oocyte surface (Figures 84–87). The progression of the sperm through the zona also involves the mobilization of acrosin, a proteolytic enzyme bound to the inner acrosomal membrane, whose bioactivity mediates the passage of the motile sperm through the zona pellucida (Figure 88) by altering chemical interactions between certain zona proteins. Accessory spermatozoa often remain on the zona surface or in association with residual corona and cumulus cells for days after fertilization.

After passage through the zona pellucida the sperm nucleus, devoid of the acrosome, enters the perivitelline space and, shortly thereafter, contacts the oocyte plasma membrane (Figure 89a, b).

Time-lapse imaging demonstrates that the tail retains active motility within the channel created in the zona matrix by the action of acrosin, and the apparent force generated by a persistent rotary pattern of tail motion may be transmitted to the sperm head to facilitate contact between the sperm nucleus and oolemma[74]. The relative strength of this force is briefly evident in some time-lapse images of the human *in vitro* fertilization process, in which a slight indentation of the oolemma occurs during the initial contact between sperm and oocyte. For example, the fertilizing spermatozoon shown in Figure 89a was observed indenting the oolemma in the region between the arrow and bar[74]. As in some other mammals, the entire tail segment is incorporated into the human oocyte during the fertilization process, as shown in Figure 89c, which is a compiled scanning laser confocal image of a newly fertilized human oocyte in which the head and tail are stained with a DNA-specific probe and a tubulin antibody, respectively.

Penetration of the sperm into the oocyte cytoplasm, the ooplasm, results in the activation of the oocyte, a general term used to describe a series of temporally and spatially coordinated molecular and cellular responses to the entrance of the male gamete. Contact between sperm and oocyte membranes (Figure 89b) is accompanied by a transient change in the polarity of the oolemma[75] that is thought to facilitate penetration and initiate the mobilization of free calcium from intracellular stores[76,77]. Increased levels of intracellular free calcium lead to the discharge of the cortical granules by an exocytotic process termed the cortical granule reaction. The discharge and hydration of cortical granule components in the perivitelline space initiates zona hardening (the zona reaction), which is an essential mechanism by which polyspermy is prevented. This is probably the case for the sperm head shown in Figure 88b that was embedded in the zona at the time of fixation, which in this instance occurred hours after the fertilizing sperm had entered the ooplasm. The 'hardening' of the zona is a normal response to penetration, but premature hardening due to biochemical or biophysical defects in zona formation, or to premature cortical granule exocytosis during preovulatory maturation, is a recognized etiology of fertilization failure in clinical IVF.

Penetration of the fertilizing spermatozoon is associated with the resumption of meiosis II, which is completed with the segregation of a half set of chromosomes (i.e. chromatids) into the second polar body. At the cytoplasmic level, oocyte activation involves the progressive development of microtubules that form an extensive network during the latter phases of the 1-cell stage[75] (Figure 90). An essential aspect of the acquisition of oocyte competence is the ability of the cytoplasm to decondense sperm DNA and transform the sperm nucleus into a male pronucleus[78]. After the completion of meiosis II, the female chromosomes decondense and become enclosed by a nascent pronuclear membrane and form the female pronucleus. The detection of two pronuclei during the 1-cell stage is the hallmark of fertilization, which in clinical IVF is confirmed by light microscopy, usually between 12 and 20 hours after insemination (Figure 91). In the human, arrays of microtubules that originate from the sperm centrosome (Figure 92) may be involved in establishing and maintaining the close proximity between the male and female pronuclei. The evolution of centrosome-associated microtubules is an early event in the fertilization process and has been observed to occur prior to significant decondensation of the sperm head (Figure 92a, b). The centrosome is located behind the basal plate and contains a proximal centriole (Figure 92c) whose duplication during the pronuclear stage provides the poles of the first (Figure 93) and all subsequent mitotic spindles. As development through the 1-cell stage progresses, portions of the opposed nuclear membranes are in direct contact or separated by a few micrometers (Figure 94).

In the human, DNA replication is initiated approximately 10–12 hours after sperm penetration (Figure 95d–h), and when completed some 10–12 hours later the opposed pronuclear membranes begin to fragment in a process termed pronuclear membrane dissolution or syngamy. Syngamy results in the first actual interaction between maternal and paternal chromosomes (Figure 95g, h) and, after pronuclear membrane dissolution, is rapidly followed by the formation of the first mitotic spindle and the segregation of replicated chromosomes into each blastomere at the first cleavage (cell) division. The normal pattern of chromatin distribution in the male and female pronucleus during DNA replication is shown in Figure 95d–h. The polarization of the chromatin to regions within each pronucleus where the nuclear membranes are opposed is of particular note in these scanning laser confocal images of newly fertilized eggs that had been stained with a DNA-specific fluorescent probe[75]. In clinical IVF, defects in the DNA replication process, the absences of pronuclear juxtaposition, and the failure of syngamy to occur in a timely fashion, or at all, have been related to early embryo demise. Although developmentally lethal, the occurrence of three pronuclei after dispermic penetration (Figure 96) does not preclude a normal syngamic process (Figures 96b, c) resulting in chromosomal segregation and cell division. Indeed, the polarized pattern of chromatin distribution in many tripronucleate embryos is indistinguishable from their normally fertilized counterparts (Figure 97a, b). Unlike the normal bipolar mitotic spindle that occurs with monospermic fertilization (Figure 97c), a tripolar spindle is common after dispermic penetration (Figure 97d), resulting in a chromosomally abnormal, triploid embryo. TEM images of a tripronucleate human embryo (Figure 96a) show the close apposition and fragmentation of the nuclear membranes during the peri-syngamic stage (Figure 96b, c).

Some clinical IVF laboratories have directed considerable attention to the characteristics of pronuclear morphology and orientation as predictive factors for embryo developmental normality and competence[48,79–82]. In particular, differences in pronuclear number, size, alignment with respect to the first and second polar bodies, and nucleolar distribution (also termed nucleolar precursor bodies (NPB; Figures 91, 95a–c, 96b)) have been cataloged during the 1-cell stage and related to embryo performance *in vitro*, chromosomal normality, and outcome after embryo transfer[48,79–81]. With this non-invasive approach to embryo evaluation, scoring systems with numerical values weighted for each characteristic have been developed to assess the relative competence of embryos within cohorts. Although the findings are controversial and by no means universally accepted at present, several recent studies have reported that pronuclear morphology and outcome are closely related[79–83]. When examined between 18 and 20 hours after insemination, embryos that are mostly likely to develop normally *in vitro* and implant after transfer are those with the following phenotype: (1) juxtaposed pronuclei of equal size which are (2) oriented in a relatively perpendicular manner with respect to the first and second polar bodies and which (3) contain NPBs that are aligned equatorially at the region of male and female pronuclear membrane opposition (e.g. Figure 91). An equatorial alignment of the NPBs may indicate that an appropriate polarized distribution of replicated DNA has occurred in each pronucleus resulting in a spatial localization of chromosomes prior to syngamy (e.g. Figure 95g, h) that facilitates their alignment on the nascent mitotic metaphase spindle and a numerically equivalent segregation into daughter blastomeres at the first cleavage division. However, differences in NPB distribution between pronuclear human embryos in the same cohort(s) are evident at the light microscopic level and can be confirmed by immunofluorescence with antibodies directed against NPB components (Figure 95a–c). If embryo selection is based on a single, time-specific inspection at the 1-cell stage, it will be important to determine if, and the extent to which, the number or spatial distribution of NPBs can change during the pronuclear stage.

Mitochondrial function and distribution at the pronuclear stage are important factors that determine embryo competence. A pronounced peri-pronuclear aggregation of mitochondria is characteristic of the 1-cell stage of human embryogenesis as shown in Figure 98a–k, which are scanning laser confocal images of pronuclear-stage embryos stained with a mitochondrion-specific fluorescent probe[56]. The sphere of mitochondria that surrounds the pronuclei largely dissipates after syngamy (Figure 98l) but redevelops around the blastomere nuclei at the 2-cell stage (Figure 98o, p). Asymmetrical peri-pronuclear accumulations have been observed in 1-cell human embryos (e.g. Figure 98d) and have been correlated with disproportionate mitochondrial segregation into blastomeres during subsequent cleavage divisions (Figure 98m, n, q–s) such that some blastomeres experience a significantly reduced capacity to generate ATP by mitochondrial respiration[56]. For blastomeres that inherit numerical mitochondrial deficits, this study reported adverse developmental consequences from slower rates of cell division to arrested cytokinesis. Cell lysis was observed when the size of the mitochondrial complement is insufficient to support cell function and integrity. With respect to understanding the underlying biological factors that influence outcome in clinical IVF, the finding that the intracytoplasmic organization of mitochondria at the pronuclear stage can have profound downstream effects on the normality of human embryogenesis demonstrates the importance of recognizing dynamic intracellular processes that characterize the earliest stages of development.

This will become especially relevant as new microscopic methods are developed for non-invasive embryo selection that include the identification of states of intracellular organization associated with high competence.

THE CLEAVAGE STAGES

The completion of the first cell division marks the beginning of the cleavage stages of preimplantation embryogenesis. The geometry of this first cleavage is usually a meridional bisection with the plane of division involving the region of the cytoplasm subjacent to the first and second polar bodies (Figures 99, 100). In clinical IVF, two characteristics considered indicative of high developmental competence are mononucleated blastomeres that are relatively equivalent in size (Figures 100a, 101a). The occurrence of multi- or micronucleated blastomeres in one or both blastomeres at the 2-cell stage is very common in embryos produced by IVF (Figure 100c) and, when detected, these embryos are eliminated for transfer or cryopreservation owing to the very high probability that they are chromosomally abnormal[84,85]. Fragmentation, the compartmentalization of an entire cell or the elimination of regions of cortical cytoplasm in small cytoplasts, is another common characteristic of early human embryos[86–89]. While fragmentation can occur between the pronuclear and 8-cell stages, it is most common after the first or second cleavage divisions. Cytoplasmic fragments occur as discrete membranous protrusions (Figure 101) or as clusters of unattached cytoplasts on the surface of blastomeres (Figures 102, 103). Several distinct fragmentation phenotypes have been identified for cultured cleavage-stage human embryos and both their pattern and severity are used in embryo competence assessment schemes[86–88]. For example, the pattern of fragmentation shown in Figure 103c usually portends early developmental failure and embryo demise, while the presence of a few small fragments localized in the cleft between blastomeres can be a normal characteristic of developmentally competent embryos (Figures 101a, b, 102). Fine structural studies show that within a cluster of fragments, some are detached while others retain cytoplasmic continuity with the subjacent blastomere[88]. Certain forms of fragmentation are developmentally benign, with most of the fragments seeming to disappear as development progresses[87]. The dynamic nature of these fragmentation patterns is demonstrated by time-lapse imaging which shows fragment resorption or lysis during embryo culture[88,90].

The second cleavage division of the human embryo is not always synchronous, and one blastomere may divide slightly ahead of the other resulting in the transient occurrence of a 3-cell embryo (Figure 104). An SEM image of a 3-cell embryo observed in cross section and which contained a relatively 'moderate' localized complement of fragments is shown in Figure 105. Prominent and typical fine structural features of normal cleavage-stage human embryos detected by TEM include numerous mitochondria, localized networks of smooth-surfaced endoplasmic reticulum and, in certain instances, fragments or their lysed membranous residues in the perivitelline space (Figure 106). Midbodies are usually located between cells that have just divided and contain a densely organized array of residual microtubules (Figure 107). In the early human embryo, midbodies may persist between blastomeres throughout cleavage and are clearly recognizable in thin sections owing to the presence of a characteristic electron-dense equatorial band (Figure 107b). Midbodies are normal structures that often serve as 'cellular sinks' for sequestering numerous regulatory proteins and enzymes which may no longer be required at high concentration, or be needed during a particular phase of the cell cycle[91].

SEM imaging of cleavage-stage human embryos reveals a remarkable geometric, ridge-like structure that is characteristic of the zona pellucida in fixed and dehydrated specimens. This organization is particularly evident in 4–8-cell embryos that resulted from intracytoplasmic sperm injection (ICSI) owing to the required removal of coronal cells prior to insemination (Figure 108). With reconstructions of serial sections, TEM analysis shows that each blastomere of a normal 4-cell human embryo contains interconnecting networks of smooth endoplasmic reticulum (Figure 109a, c). In some embryos, these networks are quite extensive, are densely packed and often extend from the pericortical cytoplasm to the vicinity of the blastomere nucleus (Figure 110). In the 4-cell human embryo, mitochondria remain largely unchanged from the undeveloped form they displayed in the ovulated oocyte (Figure 109b). However, as in previous stages, these organelles are functional in oxidative phosphorylation and produce most of the ATP required by the blastomeres during cleavage.

The normal progression of cleavage to the 8-cell stage is a critical landmark in early human development (Figures 111, 112) because it is at this time, approximately 72 hours after fertilization, that activation of the embryonic genome is thought to be largely complete, and differences in gene expression (inherited or *de novo*) of developmental significance with regard to differential cell function or fate may occur between blastomeres[92,93]. Morphological grading to identify competent embryos focuses on the 8-cell embryo and includes in the evaluations characteristics such as (1) the pattern and extent of fragmentation, if any; (2) the uniformity of cell divisions indicated by relatively equivalent blastomere size; and (3) the presence of multinucleated cells[94]. Currently, some IVF programs use a threshold number of normal-appearing (so-called 'top quality') 8-cell embryos to determine whether embryo transfer should occur on day 3 or be extended for an additional 2 or 3 days in order to assess their ability to develop to the expanded blastocyst stage[95–98]. However, it is evident from cytogenetic studies that chromosomal abnormalities can occur at relatively high frequency in 8-cell-stage embryos designated as 'top quality' on morphology alone, and one of the drawbacks of morphological assessments is evidenced by the fact that seemingly top-quality embryos containing numerical chromosomal defects can progress to the expanded blastocyst stage[99–101].

Fine structural analysis of 8-cell human embryos provides important information concerning stage-specific developmental changes indicative of normal and abnormal development. For example, blastomeres are more closely apposed than previously, with greater portions of their respective plasma membranes involved in intercellular contact and communication (Figure 112). In some embryos, one or two internal cells surrounded by blastomeres may be precursors of the inner cell mass (ICM), although this assignment is by no means certain, nor is cell fate necessarily fixed at this stage. The presence of cytoplasmic fragments between blastomeres is a common occurrence in cultured human embryos (Figure 113), and may have potentially adverse developmental effects if their number and size prevent normal intercellular contact and communication[87–89]. Embryos presumed to be normal contain mononucleated blastomeres, but the presence of bi- or multinucleated blastomeres is not uncommon (Figure 114a). Prominent features of blastomeres observed by TEM include numerous mitochondria,

networks of SER (Figures 112, 114) and midbodies (Figure 113a). Other cytoplasmic features detected in some blastomeres (but not others) are annulate lamellae, crystalloid inclusions (see below) and small stacks of Golgi saccules (Figures 112–115). The absence of a nucleus in some blastomeres is either cell-cycle related, or, if the cells are unusually small, indicative of an asymmetrical cleavage division that has generated a cytoplast. Severe fragmentation at the 4–8-cell stages is often lethal with respect to developmental viability. Fine structural analysis of affected embryos shows a pleiomorphic population of intact and lysed cytoplasts dispersed between intact blastomeres (Figure 113a). The composition of fragments can also differ with organelles such as mitochondria detected in some but not all fragments[88].

Occasionally, oocytes that resemble embryos in the early cleavage stage are aspirated from stimulated follicles during IVF procedures. In some instances, degenerative processes within the oocyte may lead to cytoplasmic compartmentalization and produce fragmentation phenotypes similar to those observed in normally fertilized cleavage-stage embryos. In other cases, the cellular compartments are of uniform diameter, mononucleated and, at the light microscopic level, morphologically similar to normal cleavage-stage embryos. Moreover, some apparently (spontaneously) activated oocytes that have never been exposed to sperm (i.e. parthenogenetic) continue to divide in culture. For example, serial paraffin sections of a human antral follicle demonstrate the presence of an apparent '4-cell' embryo, and in Figure 115a, two of the three cells shown in this section of such an embryo appear mononucleated. The finding of an activated oocyte within a sectioned antral follicle is indeed a rarity, but is not entirely unexpected as certain ovarian teratomas begin as spontaneously activated oocytes. While the oocyte shown in Figure 115a may have initiated cytokinesis, similar types of oocytes do occur in follicular aspirates. For example, TEM images of apparent 2- and 6-cell 'embryos' are shown in Figure 116a and c, respectively. TEM imaging reveals the presence of a well-formed spindle in one cell of a 2-cell parthenogenetic human embryo that was obtained in this state at aspiration (Figure 115b). Typically, cleavage-stage human embryos resulting from spontaneous activation are a mixture of mononucleated (Figure 116a) and multinucleated cells (Figure 116b). However, division to the 8-cell stage can occur (Figure

117a) and their surface features revealed by SEM are very similar to those present in their normally fertilized counterparts, including small fragments that are presumably extracellular, and blastomeres with a normal-appearing microvillus surface (Figure 117b).

THE MORULA AND BLASTOCYST STAGES

The formation of a morula around the 16-cell stage is a second essential developmental landmark in the normal progression of the human embryo through the preimplantation stages. The distinct borders between the spherical cells that characterized the earlier cleavage stages are largely lost because of a morphodynamic process termed compaction, which is a prerequisite for cavitation and blastocyst formation (see below). The compacted phenotype results from a significant elongation and flattening of the outer blastomeres (facing the zona pellucida). As contacts between opposing cells become more extensive, the outer cells can appear to surround or partially envelop subjacent (interior) blastomeres, which, by contrast, remain relatively spherical (Figure 118). As compaction progresses, tight junctions develop between the apical borders of the outer cells, permitting the formation of an effective seal that allows fluid to accumulate within the interior of the embryo during the next stage of preimplantation embryogenesis, cavitation. The formation of these junctions and the differential morphodynamic activities of cells comprising the morula begin to establish two distinct cell lineages: (1) the outer cells from which the trophoblast (also termed the trophectoderm) develops (Figures 118, 119); and (2) an inner cluster of cells from which the inner cell mass (ICM) arises. The establishment of these cell lineages is the hallmark of preimplantation embryogenesis because it is these two basic cell types that form the initial 'body' plan of the mammalian embryo[93,102]; the ICM develops into the fetus while the trophoblast forms the extraembryonic membranes and placenta. In addition, it is the trophoblast that is solely involved in the implantation process and in the biosynthesis of unique signaling and regulatory molecules and growth factors such as leptin, vascular endothelial growth factor (VEGF) and human chorionic gonadotropin (hCG), among others[103–105].

With the continued transport of fluid from the perivitelline space through the trophoblast cells by an endocytotic/exocytotic process, the blastocoel cavity progressively expands so that the distinction between the trophoblast and ICM becomes increasingly apparent (Figure 119). In this respect, and in addition to its specialized biosynthetic properties, trophoblast cells are considered a typical fluid-transporting epithelium[106]. During the early stages of blastocyst expansion, the trophoblast cells become thinner while ICM cells remain largely spherical (Figures 119, 120).

Relatively high frequencies of blastocyst development are common in contemporary clinical IVF with high-competence oocytes (> 50%), especially when culture media formulations suggested to be 'optimized' for the human embryo are used to extend in vitro development to the hatched blastocyst stage (see below)[107–109]. However, when embryos are cultured to the blastocyst stage under identical conditions (i.e. within the same microdroplet), significant morphological differences are often apparent. Differences considered to be of developmental significance include (1) total cell numbers that may be inappropriate for the stage or time in culture; (2) inappropriate cell allocation between the ICM and trophoblast; and (3) an absent, scant or disorganized ICM. These and other empirical characteristics are used to evaluate the apparent normality of development and to select blastocysts for transfer or cryopreservation[21].

Blastocysts characterized as grossly 'normal' by light microscopic criteria often display fine structural features that would seem to be inconsistent with competence (Figure 120). By TEM, presumably incompetent blastocysts display common features characterized by: (1) a disorganized or fragmented ICM containing remnants of lysed cells (black asterisk, Figure 121); and (2) trophoblast cells that are multinucleated or have no detectable nucleus (Figure 121) and are largely devoid of organelles (white asterisks, Figure 121). In some trophoblast cells, mitochondria occur in massive aggregates (arrow, Figure 121). ICM cells often contain unusual inclusions such as crystalline bodies (Figure 122a). However, whether these inclusions are indicative of a premorbid condition is unknown, as they are also detected in normal-appearing blastomeres during the cleavage stages (Figure 122b). While the blastocysts shown in Figures 120 and 121 were selected because TEM analysis (but not light microscopy) suggested developmental abnormalities, it is important to emphasize that the presence of aberrant or degenerate cells in either the ICM or trophoblast detected in selected thin sections may not be indicative of a developmentally compromised or non-viable embryo. Indeed, several reports indicate that some ICM and trophoblast cells undergo apoptotic cell death as a normal aspect of human blastocyst development[110]. Likewise, cytogenetic analysis of stage-appropriate blastocysts demonstrates that the presence of chromosomally abnormal ICM and trophoblast cells may be a typical feature of late preimplantation-stage human embryos that has no adverse consequences for normal development to birth[99–101]. It seems likely that a threshold level of abnormal or degenerating cells exists in normal blastocysts but, when exceeded, a progressive reduction in developmental competence occurs.

BLASTOCYST HATCHING – THE PRELUDE TO IMPLANTATION

The emergence of the expanded blastocyst from within the zona pellucida marks the terminal phase of preimplantation embryogenesis. The mechanism by which it escapes from the confines of the zona pellucida involves a process commonly known as 'hatching', which represents a combination of mechanical forces generated by the progressive accumulation of fluid within the blastocyst cavity and the corresponding expansion of the embryo, coupled with the release of zona lytic enzymes by certain trophoblast cells that creates a rent in a thinned zona through which the embryo emerges (Figure 123). Similar to the situation observed in other mammals (e.g. mouse and hamster), elongated filapodia expressed by a small domain of trophoblast cells have been detected in the hatching human blastocyst (Figure 124a). These filopodia are very motile and may facilitate the dissolution of the overlying zona pellucida (recently termed 'zona breakers')[111], and their absence in some fully expanded blastocysts may represent a developmentally significant defect if associated with the inability of the embryo to 'hatch'. The caliber of the rent through which the blastocyst emerges is embryo-specific and, while for some hatching seems to involve a considerable degree of zona dissolution (Figure 123b), for others, the embryo emerges from a hole that is considerably smaller (Figure 123a, c). Because defects in the hatching process will contribute to implantation failure in clinical IVF, invasive methods collectively known as 'assisted hatching' have been developed to

create an artificial hole by means of chemical, mechanical, or laser-light-induced manipulations of the zona pellucida[112]. Whether this procedure universally improves outcome in clinical IVF is controversial[112–114]. However, results with assisted hatching in clinical IVF show higher frequencies of monozygotic twinning than would be expected with natural conceptions and it has been proposed that emergence from a comparatively small opening in a normally rigid zona pellucida may be responsible[115]. However, this notion may require revision owing to the occurrence of monozygotic twinning after the transfer of zona-free blastocysts[116].

As observed by TEM, a presumably normal human blastocyst contains a well-defined ICM that is readily delineated from the surrounding trophoblast. This normal organization is especially evident when a portion of the trophoblast is expressed through the zona rent during the emergence or hatching phase (Figure 123a). At the fine structural level, the occurrence of elongated mitochondria containing well-developed cristae that fully traverse a matrix of relatively low electron density is one of the more apparent cytoplasmic changes observed in human blastocysts (Figure 124b, c). Although most mitochondria in blastocyst-stage embryos remain spherical (M1, Figure 124b), the increased occurrence of elongated forms (M2, Figure 124c) is generally thought to be an important aspect of normal development associated with elevated levels of oxidative metabolism.

The differential organization and surface architecture of the ICM and trophoblast are particularly striking when the embryo is fractured and imaged by SEM (Figures 125 and 126). As shown at low magnification in Figure 126b and at higher magnification in Figure 127, the ICM displays regional variation in surface characteristics, with some cells possessing a relatively smooth plasma membrane while others exhibit a complex surface populated by microvilli, blebs and elongated cellular processes (arrow, Figure 127, Figure 128a), the latter of which has been a suggested characteristic of a normally developed ICM. Secretory activity by the ICM may involve cells adorned by a dense and pleiotropic population of spherical bodies, cytoplasmic protrusions and blebs (asterisk, Figure 127). If secretory activity is confirmed, biochemical analysis of the blastocoelic fluid may be warranted in order to determine whether these cells produce specific or unique growth factors and other regulatory molecules that may be involved in ICM or trophoblast differentiation and function during peri-implantation stages.

The apical surface of the trophoblast displays a remarkably complex architecture composed of (1) microvilli and other cellular processes of varying diameters and lengths; (2) a pleiotropic population of secretory-like structures resident on the plasma membrane or intermingled between microvilli (Figure 128b); and (3) relatively large and bulbous paired protrusions (Figure 129, and shown in green beneath the asterisk in Figure 126). The former characteristics are consistent with cells actively engaged in the secretion of a complex mixture of adhesion molecules, growth factors and other regulatory/signaling proteins, while the latter may represent cells in the process of division (cytokinesis). Secretory features such as these would be expected to be observed by SEM in normally developing blastocysts where cell division is rapid and the expression of molecules that regulate attachment and adherence of the hatched blastocyst to endometrial epithelium is a prerequisite for the next and most important phase of early embryogenesis, implantation. In this regard, SEM remains an essential research tool for future studies of early human embryogenesis, because of its capacity to identify subtle defects or differences in surface architecture that enable or preclude stable interactions between maternal and embryonic cells that facilitate the invasive penetration of the uterus by trophoblast cells during the initial stages of implantation[117–119].

REFERENCES – SECTION TWO

1. Fauser C, Bouchard P, Hsueh A, et al. Reproductive Medicine: Molecular, Cellular and Genetic Fundamentals. New York: Parthenon Publishing, 2003

2. Rinaudo P, Schultz R. Effects of embryo culture on global pattern of gene expression in preimplantation mouse embryos. Reproduction 2004; 128: 301–11

3. Van Blerkom J. Developmental failure in human reproduction associated with chromosomal abnormalities and cytoplasmic pathologies in meiotically mature oocytes. In Van Blerkom J, ed. The Biological Basis of Early Human Reproductive Failure. Oxford: Oxford University Press, 1994: 283–326

4. Hall S. The good egg. Discover 2004; 25: 30–9

5. von Baer C. De ovi Mammalium et Hominis Genesi. Lipsiae; 1827

6. van Beneden E. La maturation de l'oeuf, la fecondation et les premieres phases du developpement des mammiferes d' après recherches faites chez le lapin. Bull Acad Belg Classe Sci 1875; 40: 686–9

7. Hertwig O. Beitrage zur Kenntniss der Bildung, Befruchtung und Theilung des thierischen Eies. Morph Jarbuch 1876; 1: 347–434

8. Haeckel E. The Evolution of Man: Human Embryology or Ontogeny, 5th edn. New York: Peter Eckler Publisher, 1906

9. Wilmut I, Schnieke A, McWhir J, et al. Viable offspring derived from fetal and adult mammalian cells. Nature 1997; 385: 810–13

10. Kono T, Obata Y, Wu Q, et al. Birth of parthenogenetic mice that can develop to adulthood. Nature 2004; 428: 860–4

11. Hubner K, Fuhrmann G, Christenson L, et al. Derivation of oocytes from mouse embryonic stem cells. Science 2003; 300: 1251–6

12. Geijsen N, Horoschak M, Kim K, et al. Derivation of embryonic germ cells and male gametes from embryonic stem cells. Nature 2004; 427: 148–54

13. Silber S. Genetics of male infertility: evolution of the X and Y chromosome and transmission of male infertility to future generations. In Van Blerkom J, Gregory L, eds. Essential IVF: Basic Research and Clinical Applications. Boston: Kluwer Academic Publishers, 2004: 111–49

14. Cummins J. Can and should human embryos be 'rescued' from developmental demise? Methods and biological basis. In Van Blerkom J, Gregory L, eds. Essential IVF: Basic Research and Clinical Applications. Boston: Kluwer Academic Publishers, 2004: 555–75

15. Verlinsky Y, Kuliev A. An Atlas of Preimplantation Genetic Diagnosis. New York: Parthenon Publishing, 2000

16. Edwards R. Causes of early embryonic loss in human pregnancy. Hum Reprod 1986; 1: 185–98

17. Gregory L. Perifollicular vascularity: a marker of follicular heterogeneity and oocyte competence and a predictor of implantation in assisted conception cycles. In Van Blerkom J, Gregory L, eds. Essential IVF: Basic Research and Clinical Applications. Boston: Kluwer Academic Publishers, 2004: 59–79

18. Gerris J. Reducing the number of embryos to transfer after IVF/ICSI. In Van Blerkom J, Gregory L, eds. Essential IVF: Basic Research and Clinical Applications. Boston: Kluwer Academic Publishers, 2004: 505–54

19. Van Blerkom J, Henry G. Oocyte dysmorphism and aneuploidy in meiotically-mature human oocytes

after controlled ovarian stimulation. Hum Reprod 1992; 7: 379–90

20. Veeck L. An Atlas of Human Gametes and Conceptuses. New York: Parthenon Publishing, 1999

21. Veeck L, Zaninovic N, eds. An Atlas of Human Blastocysts. New York: Parthenon Publishing, 2003

22. Hnida C, Engenheiro E, Ziebe S. Computer-controlled, multilevel, morphometric analysis of blastomere size as biomarker of fragmentation and multinuclearity in human embryos. Hum Reprod 2004; 19: 288–93

23. Motta P, Makabe S. An Atlas of Menopausal Aging. New York: Parthenon Publishing, 2003

24. Gosden R, Clarke H, Miller D. Female gametogenesis. In Fauser BC, et al., eds. Reproductive Medicine: Molecular, Cellular and Genetic Fundamentals. New York: Parthenon Publishing, 2003: 365–80

25. Maro B, Johnson M, Webb M, Flach G. Mechanism of polar body formation in the mouse oocyte: an interaction between the chromosomes, the cytoskeleton and the plasma membrane. J Embryol Exp Morphol 1986; 92: 11–32

26. Van Blerkom J, Bell H. Regulation of development in the fully grown mouse oocyte: chromosome-mediated temporal and spatial differentiation of the cytoplasm and plasma membrane. J Embryol Exp Morphol 1986; 93: 213–38

27. Pellicer F, Andreo B, Arnal F, et al. Mechanisms of nondisjunction in human female meioses: the coexistence of two modes of malsegregation evidenced by the karyotyping of 1397 in-vitro unfertilized oocytes. Hum Reprod 2002; 17: 2134–45

28. Pellestor F, Anahory T, Hamamah S. The chromosomal analysis of human oocytes. An overview of established procedures. Hum Reprod Update 2005; 11: 15–32

29. Eichenlaub-Ritter U, Sun F. Maternal age and oocyte competence. In Van Blerkom J, Gregory L, eds. Essential IVF: Basic Research and Clinical Applications. Boston: Kluwer Academic Publishers, 2004: 201–30

30. Obata Y, Kono T. Maternal primary imprinting is established at a specific time for each gene throughout oocyte growth. J Biol Chem 2002; 277: 5285–9

31. Moore T, Haig D. Genomic imprinting in mammalian development: a parental tug-of-war. Trends Genet 1991; 7: 45–9

32. Young L, Sinclair K, Wilmut I. Large offspring syndrome in cattle and sheep. Rev Reprod 1998; 3: 155–63

33. Yojng L, Ferandes K, McEnvoy T, et al. Epigenetic changes in IGF2R is associated with fetal overgrowth after sheep embryo culture. Nat Genet 2001; 27: 153–4

34. Sinclair K, Young L, Wilmut I, McEvoy T. In-utero overgrowth in ruminants following embryo culture: lessons from mice and a warning to men. Hum Reprod 2000; 15: 68–86

35. Niemitz E, Feinberg A. Epigenetics and assisted reproductive technology: a call for investigation. Am J Hum Genet 2004; 74: 599–609

36. Moll A, Imhof S, Cruysberg J, Schouten-van Meeteren A. Incidence of retinoblastoma in children born after in-vitro fertilization. Lancet 2003; 361: 309–10

37. Eppig J, Schultz R, O'Brien M, Chesnel F. Relationship between the developmental programs controlling nuclear and cytoplasmic maturation of mouse oocytes. Dev Biol 1994; 164: 1–9

38. Ducibella T, Buetow J. Competence to undergo normal fertilization-induced cortical activation develops after metaphase I of meiosis in mouse oocytes. Dev Biol 1994; 165: 95–104

39. Moor R, Dai Y, Lee C, Fulka J. Oocyte maturation and embryonic failure. Hum Reprod Update 1998; 4: 223–36

40. Cavilla J, Hartshorne G. Oocyte competence and in vitro maturation. In Van Blerkom J, Gregory L, eds. Essential IVF: Basic Research and Clinical Applications. Boston: Kluwer Academic Publishers, 2004: 241–71

41. Chui D, Pugh N, Walker S, et al. Follicular vascularity – the predictive value of transvaginal power Doppler ultrasonography in an in vitro fertilization programme: a preliminary study. Hum Reprod 1997; 12: 191–6

42. Van Blerkom J, Antczak M, Schrader R. The developmental potential of the human oocyte is related to the dissolved oxygen content of follicular fluid: association with vascular endothelial growth factor and perifollicular blood flow characteristics. Hum Reprod 1997; 12: 1047–55

43. Gregory L. Peri-follicular vascularity: a marker of follicular heterogeneity and oocyte competence and a predictor of implantation in assisted conception cycles. In Van Blerkom J, Gregory L, eds. Essential IVF: Basic Research and Clinical Applications. Boston: Kluwer Academic Publishers, 2004: 59–79

44. Coulam C, Goodman C, Rinehart J. Color Doppler indices of follicular blood flow as predictors of pregnancy after in vitro fertilization and embryo transfer. Hum Reprod 1999; 14: 1979–82

45. Plachot M. Genetic analysis of the oocyte – a review. Placenta 2003; 24 (Suppl 2): S66–9

46. Van Blerkom J. Follicular influences on oocyte and embryo competence. In DeJonge C, Barratt C, eds. Assisted Reproductive Technology: Accomplishments and New Horizons. Cambridge: Cambridge University Press, 2002: 81–105

47. Gaulden M. The enigma of Down syndrome and other trisomic conditions. Mutat Res 1992; 269: 69–88

48. Scott L. The biological basis of oocyte and embryo competence: morphodynamic criteria for embryo selection in in-vitro fertilization. In Van Blerkom J, Gregory L, eds. Essential IVF: Basic Research and Clinical Applications. Boston: Kluwer Academic Publishers, 2004: 331–76

49. Eppig J. Oocyte control of ovarian follicular development and function in mammals. Reproduction 2001; 122: 829–38

50. Albertini D, Barrett S. Oocyte–somatic cell communication. Reproduction (Suppl) 2003; 61: 49–54

51. Albertini D. Oocyte–granulosa cell interactions. In Van Blerkom J, Gregory L, eds. Essential IVF: Basic Research and Clinical Applications. Boston: Kluwer Academic Publishers, 2004: 43–58

52. Antczak M, Van Blerkom J. Oocyte influences on early development: the regulatory proteins leptin and STAT3 are polarized in mouse and human oocytes and differentially distributed within the cells of the preimplantation stage embryo. Mol Hum Reprod 1997; 3: 1067–86

53. Van Blerkom J, Motta P. The Cellular Basis of Mammalian Reproduction. Baltimore: Urban and Schwarzenberg, 1979

54. Van Blerkom J, Davis P, Lee J. ATP content of human oocytes and developmental potential and outcome after in-vitro fertilization and embryo transfer. Hum Reprod 1995; 10: 415–24

55. Van Blerkom J. The role of mitochondria in human oogenesis and preimplantation embryogenesis: engines of metabolism, ionic regulation and developmental competence. Reproduction 2004; 128: 269–80

56. Van Blerkom J, Davis P, Alexander S. Differential mitochondrial inheritance between blastomeres in cleavage stage human embryos: determination of the pronuclear stage and relationship to micotubular organization, ATP content and developmental competence. Hum Reprod 2000; 15: 2621–33

57. Reynier P, May-Panloup P, Chretien M, et al. Mitochondrial DNA content affects the fertilizability of human oocytes. Mol Hum Reprod 2001; 7: 425–9

58. Motta P, Nottola S, Makabe S, Heyn R. Mitochondrial morphology in human fetal and adult female germ cells. Hum Reprod 2000; 15 (Suppl 2): 129–47

59. Van Blerkom J. Occurrence and developmental consequences of aberrant cellular organization in meiotically mature human oocytes after exogenous ovarian hyperstimulation. J Electron Microscop Tech 1990; 16: 324–46

60. Meriano J, Alexis J, Visram-Zaver S, et al. Tracking of oocyte dysmorphisms for ICSI patients may prove relevant to the outcome in subsequent patient cycles. Hum Reprod 2001; 16: 2118–23

61. Van Blerkom J, Davis P, Merriam J. The developmental ability of human oocytes penetrated at the germinal vesicle stage after insemination in vitro. Hum Reprod 1994; 9: 697–708

62. Verlinsky U, Kuliev A. Genetic diagnosis of metaphase II oocytes. In Van Blerkom J, Gregory L, eds. Essential IVF: Basic Research and Clinical Applications. Boston: Kluwer Academic Publishers, 2004: 231–40

63. Tesarik J. Calcium signalling in human oocytes and embryos: two-store model revival. Hum Reprod 2002; 17: 2948–9

64. Dumollard R, Hammar K, Porterfield M, et al. Mitochondrial respiration and Ca^{2+} waves are linked during fertilisation and meiosis completion. Development 2003; 130: 683–92

65. Otsuki J, Okada A, Morimoto K, et al. The relationship between pregnancy outcome and smooth endoplasmic reticulum clusters in MII human oocytes. Hum Reprod 2004; 19: 1591–7

66. Ozil J, Huneau D. Activation of rabbit oocytes: the impact of the Ca2+ signal regime on development. Development 2001; 128: 917–28

67. Battaglia D, Goodwin P, Klein N, et al. Influence of maternal age on meiotic spindle assembly in oocytes from naturally cycling women. Mol Hum Reprod 1996; 11: 2217–22

68. Van Blerkom J, Davis P, Alexander S. Delayed evolution of a sperm-derived mitotic spindle in the absence of male pronuclear formation in apparently unfertilized human oocytes. Reprod BioMed Online 2004; 8: 454–9

69. Wang W, Meng L, Hackett R, et al. Developmental ability of human oocytes with or without birefringent spindles imaged by Polscope before insemination. Hum Reprod 2001; 16: 1464–8

70. Van Blerkom J, Davis P, Alexander S. Inner mitochondrial membrane potential cytoplasmic ATP content and free calcium levels in metaphase II mouse oocytes. Hum Reprod 2003; 18: 2429–40

71. Jones A, Van Blerkom J, Davis P, Toledo A. Cryopreservation of metaphase II human oocytes effects mitochondrial inner membrane potential: implications for developmental competence. Hum Reprod 2004; 19: 1861–6

72. Aw T-Y. Intracellular compartmentalization of organelles and gradients of low molecular weight species. Int Rev Cytol 2000; 192: 223–53

73. Van Blerkom J, Henry G. Dispermic fertilization of human oocytes. J Electron Microsc Tech 1991; 17: 437–49

74. Van Blerkom J, Davis P, Merriam J, Sinclair J. Nuclear and cytoplasmic dynamics of sperm penetration, pronuclear formation, and microtubule organization during fertilization and early preimplantation development in the human. Hum Reprod Update 1995; 1: 429–61

75. Gianaroli L, Tosti E, Magli C, et al. Fertilization current in the human oocyte. Mol Reprod Dev 1994; 38: 209–14

76. Sousa M, Barros A, Tesarik J. The role of ryanodine-sensitive Ca^{2+} store in the Ca^{2+} oscillation machine of human oocytes. Mol Hum Reprod 1996; 2: 699–708

77. Van Blerkom J, Davis P, Alexander S. Inner mitochondrial membrane potential, cytoplasmic ATP content and free Ca (2+) levels in metaphase II mouse oocytes. Hum Reprod 2003; 18: 2429–40

78. Tesarik J. Developmental failure during the preimplantation period of human embryogenesis. In Van Blerkom J, ed. The Biological Basis of Early Human Reproductive Failure. Oxford: Oxford University Press, 1994: 327–44

79. Garello C, Baker H, Rai J, et al. Pronuclear orientation, polar body placement, and embryo quality after intracytoplasmic sperm injection and in vitro fertilization: further evidence for polarity by single human preimplantation embryos. Hum Reprod 1999; 14: 2588–95

80. Tesarik J, Greco E. The probability of abnormal preimplantation development can be predicted by a single static observation on pronuclear stage morphology. Hum Reprod 1999; 14: 1318–23

81. Scott L, Alvero R, Leondires M, et al. The morphology of human pronuclear embryos is positively related to blastocyst development and implantation. Hum Reprod 2000; 15: 2394–403

82. Gianaroli L, Magli M, Ferraretti A, et al. Pronuclear morphology and chromosomal abnormalities as scoring criteria for embryo selection. Fertil Steril 2003; 80: 341–9

83. Balaban B, Yakin K, Urman B, et al. Pronuclear morphology predicts embryo development and chromosome constitution. Reprod BioMed Online 2004; 8: 695–700

84. Hardy K, Winston R, Handyside A. Binucleate blastomeres in preimplantation human embryos in vitro: failure of cytokinesis during early cleavage. J Reprod Fertil 1993; 98: 549–58

85. Meriano J, Clark C, Cadesky K, et al. Binucleated and micronucleated blastomeres in embryos derived from human assisted reproduction cycles. Reprod BioMed Online 2004; 9: 511–20

86. Antczak M, Van Blerkom J. Temporal and spatial aspects of fragmentation in early human embryos: possible effects on developmental competence and association with the differential elimination of regulatory proteins from polarized domains. Hum Reprod 1999; 14: 429–47

87. Alikani M, Cohen J, Tomkin G, et al. Human embryo fragmentation in vitro and its implications for pregnancy and implantation. Fertil Steril 1999; 71: 836–42

88. Van Blerkom J, Davis P, Alexander S. Human embryo fragmentation: a multifaceted microscopic, biochemical and experimental study of fragmentation in early human preimplantation stage embryos. Hum Reprod 2001; 16: 719–29

89. Van Blerkom J. The enigma of fragmentation in early human embryos: possible causes and clinical relevance. In Van Blerkom J, Gregory L, eds. Essential IVF: Basic Research and Clinical Applications. Boston: Kluwer Academic Publishers, 2004: 377–422

90. Hardarson T, Lofman C, Coull G, et al. Internalization of cellular fragments in a human embryo: time-lapse recordings. Reprod BioMed Online 2002; 5: 36–8

91. Skop A, Liu H, Yates J, et al. Dissection of the mammalian midbody proteome reveals conserved cytokinesis mechanisms. Science 2004; 305: 61–6

92. Braude P, Bolton V, Moore S. Human gene expression first occurs between the four- and eight cell stage of preimplantation development. Nature 1989; 332: 459–61

93. Edwards R. Genetics of polarity in mammalian embryos. Reprod BioMed Online 2005; 11: 104–14

94. Rienzi L. Significance of morphological attributes of the early embryo. Reprod BioMed Online 2005; 10: 669–81

95. Borini A. Predictive factors for embryo implantation potential. Reprod BioMed Online 2005; 10: 653–68

96. Rienzi L, Ubaldi F, Iacobelli M, et al. Day 3 embryo transfer with combined evaluation at the pronuclear and cleavage stages compares favorably with day 5 blastocyst transfer. Hum Reprod 2002; 17: 1852–5

97. Racowsky C, Jackson K, Cekleniak N, et al. The number of eight-cell embryos is a key determinant for selecting day 3 or day 5 transfer. Fertil Steril 2000; 73: 558–64

98. Gerris J, De Neubourg D, Mangelschots K, et al. Elective single day 3 embryo transfer halves the twinning rate without decrease in the ongoing preg-

nancy rate of an IVF/ICSI programme. Hum Reprod 2002; 17: 626–31

99. Sandalinas M, Sadowy S, Alikani M, et al. Developmental ability of chromosomally abnormal human embryos to develop to the blastocyst stage. Hum Reprod 2001; 16: 1954–8

100. Derhaag J, Coonen E, Bras M, et al. Chromosomally abnormal cells are not selected for the extra-embryonic compartment of the human preimplantation embryo at the blastocyst stage. Hum Reprod 2003; 18: 2565–74

101. Evsikov S, Verlinsky Y. Moasicism in the inner cell mass of human blastocysts. Hum Reprod 1998; 13: 3151–5

102. Gardner R. The early blastocyst is bilaterally symmetrical and its axis of symmetry is aligned with the animal–vegetal axis of the zygote in the mouse. Development 1997; 124: 289–301

103. Emilani S. Embryo–maternal interactive factors regulating the implantation process: implications in assisted reproductive treatment. Reprod BioMed Online 2005; 10: 527–40

104. Krussel J, Behr B, Hirchenhain J, et al. Expression of vascular endothelial growth factor mRNA in human preimplantation embryos derived from tripronucleate zygotes. Fertil Steril 2000; 74: 1220–6

105. Cervero A, Horcajadas J, Dominguez F, Pellicer A, Simon C. Leptin system in embryo development and implantation: a protein in search of a function. Reprod BioMed Online 2005; 10: 217–23

106. Flemming T, Johnson M. From egg to epithelium. Ann Rev Cell Biol 1988; 4: 459–86

107. Behr B. Blastocyst culture and transfer. Hum Reprod 1999; 14: 5–6

108. Biggers J. Fundamentals of the design of culture media that support human preimplantation development. In Van Blerkom J, Gregory L, eds. Essential IVF: Basic Research and Clinical Applications. Boston: Kluwer Academic Publishers, 2004: 291–332

109. Veiga A, Torello J, Boison I, et al. Blastocyst transfer update: pros and cons. In Van Blerkom J, Gregory L,

eds. Essential IVF: Basic Research and Clinical Applications. Boston: Kluwer Academic Publishers, 2004: 423–40

110. Hardy K. Apoptosis in the human embryo. Rev Reprod 1999; 4: 125–34

111. Sathananthan H, Menezes J, Gunasheela S. Mechanics of human blastocyst hatching in vitro. Reprod BioMed Online 2003; 7: 228–34

112. Wright G, Jones A. Assisted hatching in clinical IVF. In Van Blerkom J, Gregory L, eds. Essential IVF: Basic Research and Clinical Applications. Boston: Kluwer Academic Publishers, 2004: 441–63

113. Edi-Osagie E, Hooper L, Seif M. The impact of assisted hatching on live birth rates and outcomes of assisted conception: a systematic review. Hum Reprod 2003; 18: 1828–35

114. Edi-Osagie E, Hooper L, McGinlay P, Seif M. Effect(s) of assisted hatching on assisted conception (IVF & ICSI). Cochrane Database Syst Rev 2003; 4: CD001894

115. Sills E, Tucker M, Palermo G. Assisted reproductive technologies and monozygous twins: implications for future study and clinical practice. Twin Res 2000; 3: 217–23

116. Frankfurter D, Trimarchi J, Hackett R, Meng L, Keefe D. Monozygotic pregnancies from transfers of zona-free blastocysts. Fertil Steril 2004; 82: 483–5

117. Imakawa K, Chang K, Christenson R. Pre-implantation conceptus and maternal uterine communications: molecular events leading to successful implantation. J Reprod Dev 2004; 50: 155–69

118. Hoozemans D, Schats R, Lambalk C, et al. Human embryo implantation: current knowledge and clinical implications in assisted reproductive technology. Reprod BioMed Online 2004; 9: 692–715

119. Emiliani S, Delbaere A, Devreker F, Englert Y. Embryo–maternal interactive factors regulating the implantation process: implications in assisted reproductive treatment. Reprod BioMed Online 2005; 10: 527–40

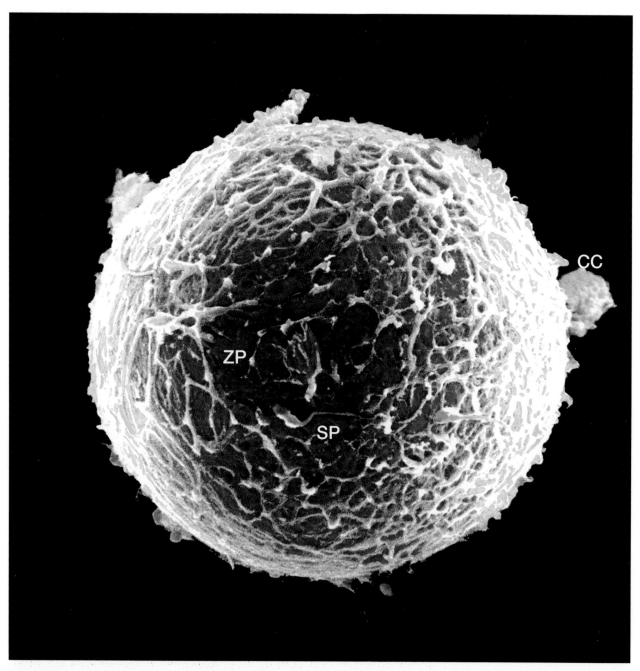

Figure 84 After fixation and preparation for SEM, the surface of the human zona pellucida (ZP) displays a characteristic architecture denoted by a geometric-like pattern of ridges. Accessory sperm (SP) are those that have attached to the zona surface but have either not penetrated the matrix or are unable to penetrate owing to 'hardening' of the zona (the zona reaction) that occurs shortly after fertilization as a result of cortical granule exocytosis. Premature hardening of the zona in mature human oocytes, i.e. prior to insemination, may be a cause of fertilization failure if most or all oocytes are affected. This phenomenon has been suggested to be a cause of infertility for some women that can be treated with *in vitro* fertilization (IVF) techniques such as the mechanical insertion of a sperm into the oocyte by means of a procedure termed intracytoplasmic sperm injection (ICSI). There are also instances in clinical IVF where no sperm are observed on the surface of the zona, despite motility and morphology characteristics that are consistent with normal male gametes. In these situations, it has been suggested that defects in sperm- or zona-binding receptors may be proximal causes of fertilization failure. CC, residual corona radiata cell

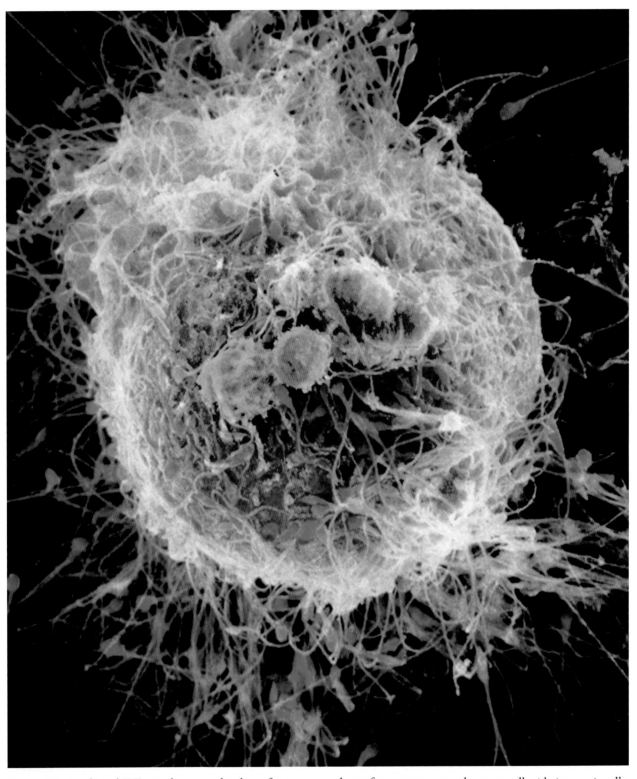

Figure 85 In clinical IVF, attachment or binding of massive numbers of spermatozoa to the zona pellucida is occasionally observed, as is shown in this SEM image of an affected zona in a 4-cell embryo some 48 hours after insemination. In most cases, not all oocytes from the same cohort inseminated under the same conditions are affected, which indicates that molecular heterogeneity in the ability of the zona to bind sperm exists and is oocyte-specific. Oocytes in which massive sperm attachment occurs are immediately identifiable in culture because the densely attached population of motile sperm causes the oocyte to rotate. If fertilized, these oocytes are usually chromosomally abnormal as a result of polyspermy, the penetration of the ooplasm by two or more spermatozoa

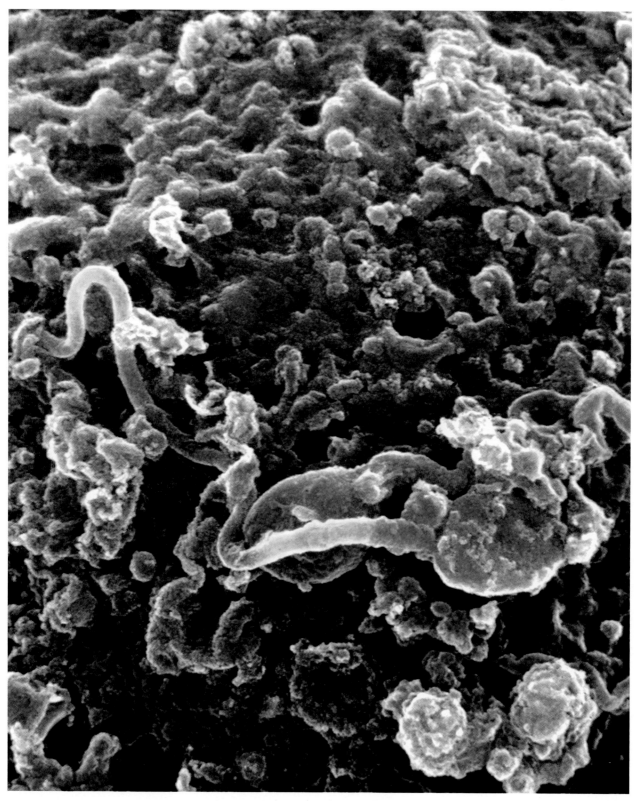

Figure 86 The interactions between sperm and the zona pellucida are shown in this high-magnification SEM image. Here, the detection of zona matrix material on the head region of the sperm suggests that this gamete had undergone the acrosome reaction and, with the putative release of acrosin, was in the initial stages of digesting a path into the zona when fixed for microscopy

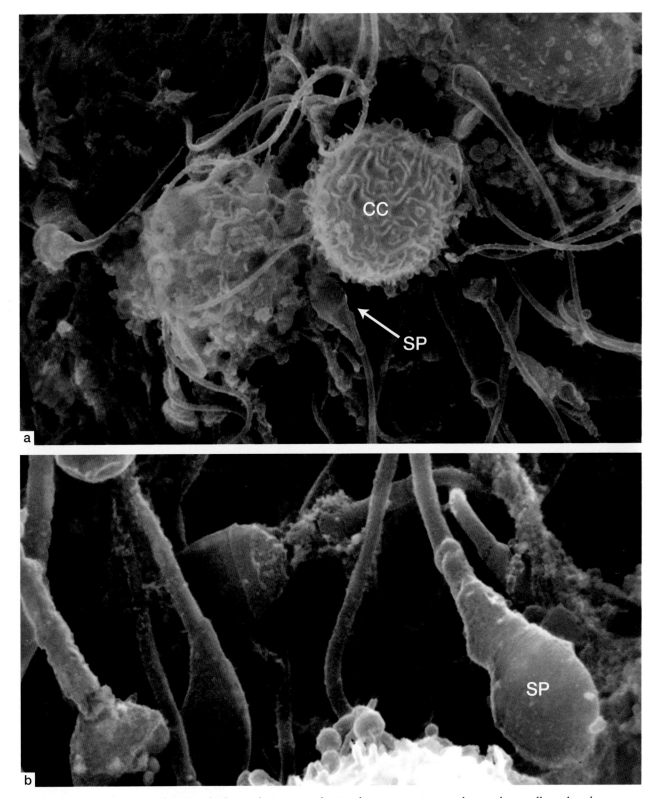

Figure 87 In conventional IVF, which involves co-incubation between sperm and granulosa cell enclosed oocytes, accessory spermatozoa attached to cells of the cumulus oophorus (CC) are always present, as shown in this SEM image (a) of a human oocyte fixed 48 hours after insemination. As the surface of the zona pellucida is imaged in this oocyte (b), both accessory sperm that can no longer penetrate the zona pellucida as well as the seemingly porous structure of this acellular coat are apparent

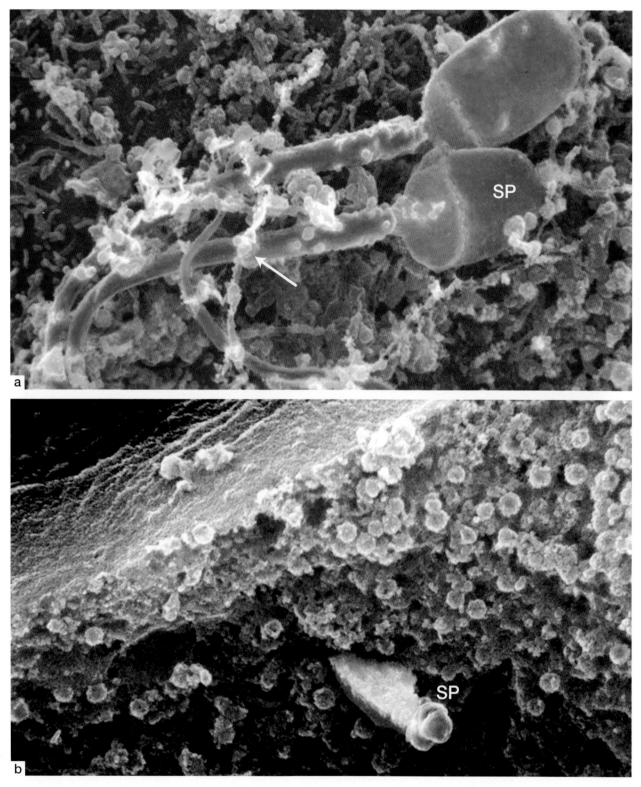

Figure 88 These SEM images reveal subtle details of sperm morphology when in proximity to the oocyte plasma membrane (oolemma). Digestion of the zona pellucida by the sperm-derived lytic enzyme acrosin produces fine fibrils through which the head of the sperm passes (a). After fertilization, the exocytosis of cortical granules into the perivitelline space and the diffusion of their contents into the zona pellucida induce a physical–chemical change in the zona pellucida resulting in a hardening of this coat and immobilization of any sperm in the process of penetration. The head of an immobilized sperm is shown in (b)

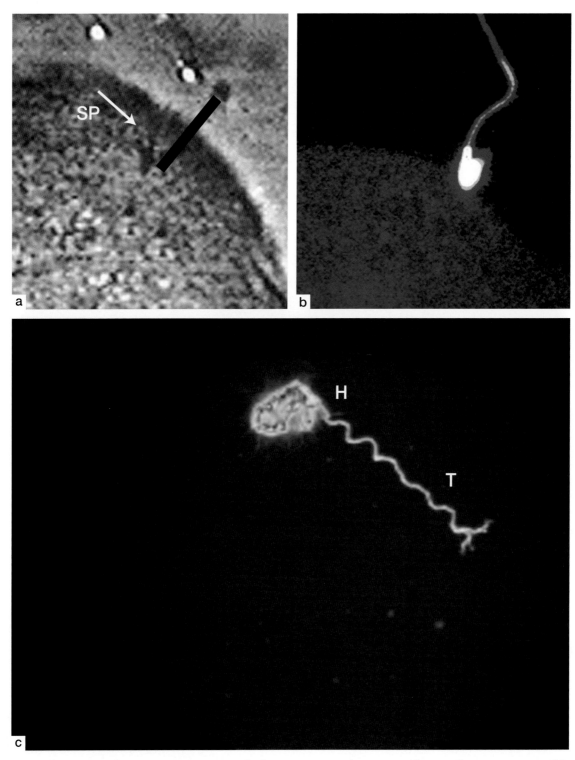

Figure 89 The process of sperm penetration into the human oocyte is best imaged by time-lapse microscopy. (a) is one image from a sequence of frames taken over several minutes after the fertilizing sperm was observed on the oolemma. The arrow-shaped sperm head, which is located between the bar and the arrow, seems to indent the oolemma. Playback of this sequence showed active rotary motility of the tail segment in the perivitelline space and inner portion of the zona pellucida. (b) and (c) are scanning laser confocal images of penetrated human oocytes in which the sperm DNA and tail microtubules were stained with specific fluorescent probes. The moment of sperm attachment to the oolemma is shown in a 5-μm digital section in (b). In the human, the entire sperm tail is incorporated into the ooplasm during the fertilization process. The appearance of a fully incorporated sperm from head (H) to tail (T) is shown in (c). This reconstructed digital image of a penetrated oocyte was produced by compiling multiple serial images taken at 2-μm intervals

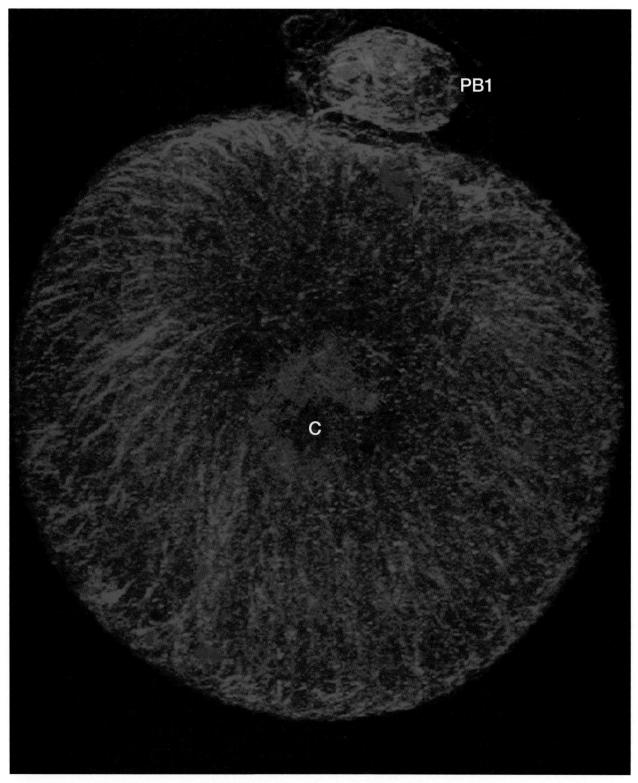

Figure 90 The activation of the human oocyte initiated by the fertilizing sperm is accompanied by major changes in cytoplasmic structure and function. The development of an extensive cytoplasmic network of microtubules is one of the more evident and developmentally critical changes, as shown in this scanning laser confocal fluorescent microscopic image of an experimentally activated MII human oocyte stained with anti-tubulin antibodies for microtubules (red) and with a DNA-specific fluorescent probe for chromosomes (C, blue). The absence of such a network after experimental activation or sperm penetration in mature human oocytes has been associated with fertilization failure and developmental arrest at the 1-cell stage

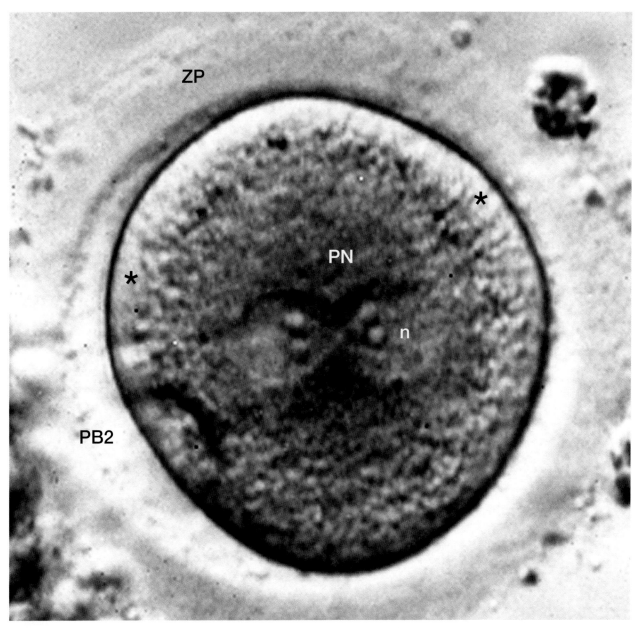

Figure 91 Stage-specific changes in cytoplasmic organization and function in pronuclear stage embryos are currently thought to be critical determinants of embryo competence during both the pre- and postimplantation phases of human embryogenesis. This light microscopic image of a human pronuclear egg shows the following aspects of cytoplasmic organization that have been suggested to be associated with developmental competence: (1) an equatorial alignment of nucleoli (n, also termed nucleolar precursor bodies); (2) pronuclear orientation that is relatively perpendicular to the first and second polar bodies (PB2); (3) a region of cortical translucency (asterisks) giving this region a halo-like appearance; and (4) an hourglass appearance of the juxtaposed pronuclei (PN) indicating that nuclear membrane dissolution, a prerequisite for the mixing of the maternal and paternal chromosomes, or syngamy is taking place. This particular pronuclear embryo was conceived by conventional IVF and developed into a normal infant

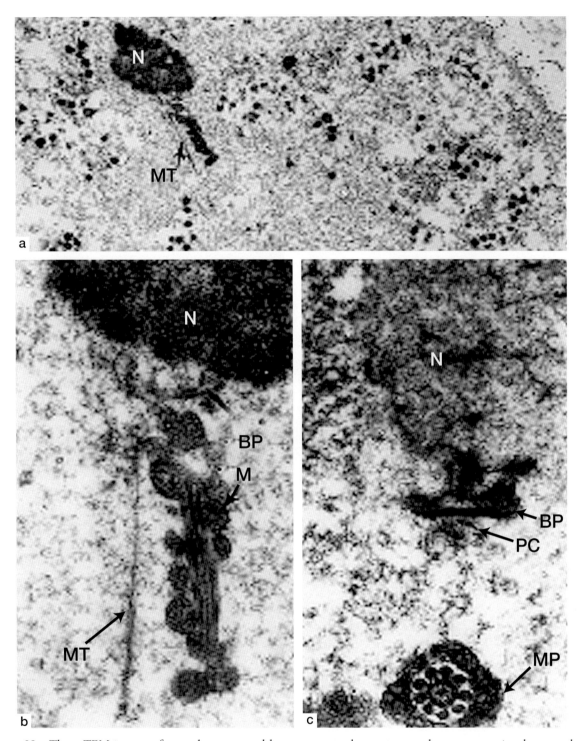

Figure 92 These TEM images of a newly penetrated human oocyte demonstrate early sperm-associated events that are critical for normal embryogenesis. While sperm DNA is beginning to decondense, the arrow-like shape of the head is still apparent some 2 hours after penetration. The plasma membrane that formerly surrounded mitochondria in the midpiece (MP) region has fully disappeared and elongated microtubules (MT) emanating from the centrosomal region are evident (a, b). While sperm mitochondria retain their characteristic helical organization in the midpiece (M, b) that lies beneath the basal plate (BP, b, c), they will become disorganized and be eliminated from the cytoplasm by maternal factors that target paternal mitochondria for destruction. This targeted molecular destruction ensures the continuity of maternal inheritance of mitochondria and mitochondrial DNA

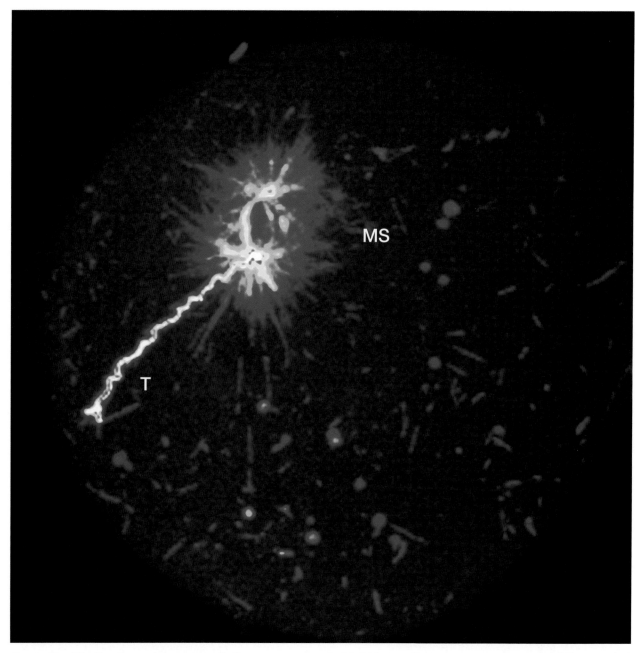

Figure 93 The first human mitotic spindle forms approximately 20–24 hours after sperm penetration. This fully compiled scanning laser confocal fluorescent image of an anti-tubulin-stained late pronuclear-stage human embryo shows the development of spindle microtubules (MS) as well as the remnant of the fully incorporated sperm tail (T)

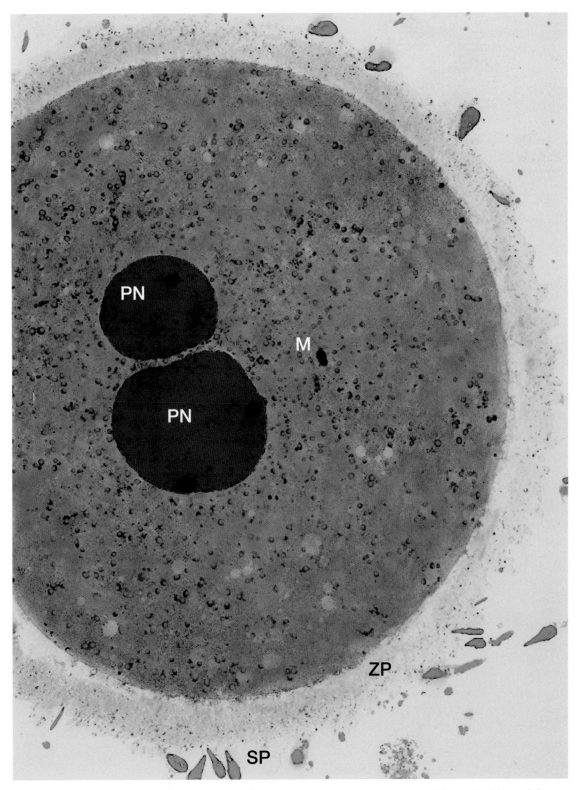

Figure 94 After conventional IVF, decondensation of maternal chromosomes and paternal (sperm) DNA and their separate enclosure by a pronuclear membrane is evident as early as 8 hours after penetration. This TEM image of a 10-hour-old human embryo shows an early stage of pronuclear evolution that is characterized by a male pronucleus (PN; lower right) that is slightly smaller in diameter than its female counterpart, and by the close opposition of the pronuclei in the approximate center of the oocyte. Despite the occurrence of numerous accessory spermatozoa (SP) on or within the zona pellucida, the presence of a single male pronucleus is evidence of normal (monospermic) penetration indicating the oocyte's ability to mount an effective block to polyspermic penetration. This is further demonstrated by the absence of cortical granules, which were discharged by exocytosis shortly after the fertilizing spermatozoon contacted the oocyte plasma membrane

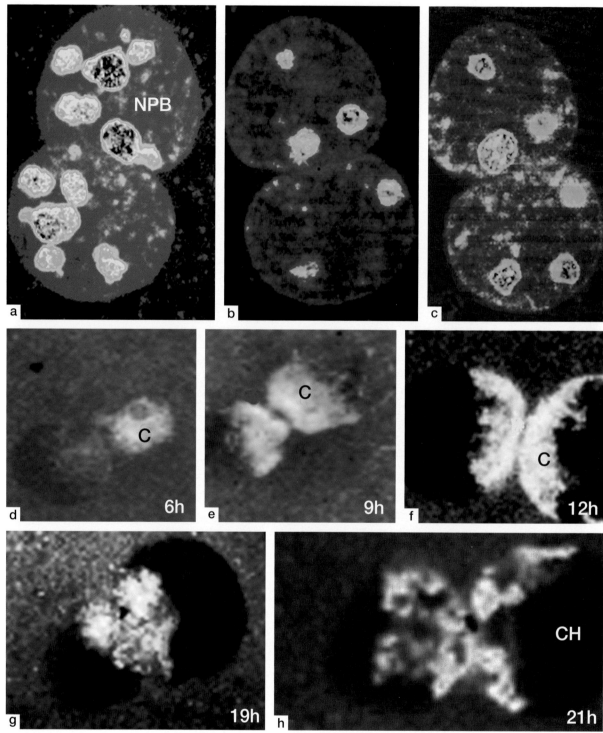

Figure 95 The number and relative position of nucleolar precursor bodies (NPB) is one of the features of early pronuclear-stage human embryos suggested to indicate normal developmental competence after IVF. (a–c) are scanning laser confocal fluorescent images of three sibling pronuclear embryos stained with anti-NPB antibodies at 22 hours after insemination. The fluorescent images show NPB characteristics to be embryo specific, i.e. they can vary significantly between embryos in the same cohort. Whether NPB number and distribution within each pronucleus are strong indicators of competence remains controversial. (d–h) show the progressive polarization of replicating pronuclear chromatin (DNA, C) to regions where the male and female pronuclei are in direct opposition. As a result, when pronuclear membrane dissolution begins (19 hours in the embryo shown in g) as a prelude to the mixing of maternal and paternal chromosomes at syngamy (CH, 21 hours after insemination in the embryo shown in h), the masses of paternal and maternal DNA are already juxtaposed. Abnormalities in this polarized distribution have been detected in pronuclear embryos produced by IVF and associated with significant numerical chromosomal defects in subsequent blastomeres and demise during the preimplantation stages

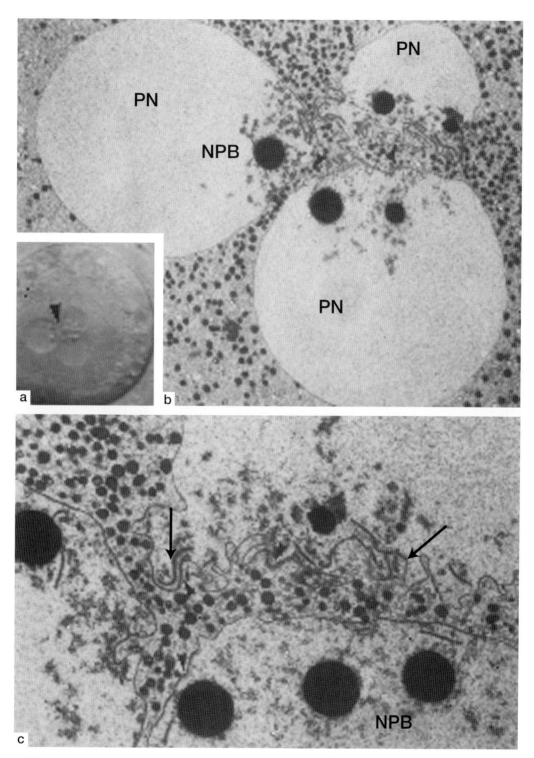

Figure 96 Polyspermy, the penetration of the mature oocyte by more than one spermatozoon, is one of the unfortunate and relatively uncontrollable aspects of conventional clinical IVF. Although frequencies of polyspermy have been reduced considerably as newer techniques of sperm preparation have been introduced that require fewer sperm for insemination, tripronucleate (PN) embryos resulting from dispermic penetration still occur (a). Often, the early *in vitro* development of tripronucleate embryos, which are chromosomally triploid, is indistinguishable from that of their normally fertilized siblings and they undergo pronuclear juxtaposition and membrane dissolution at the same time as normally fertilized eggs. (b) and (c) are TEM images of pronuclear membrane dissolution in a tripronucleate human embryo. The pattern of fragmentation of the pronuclear membranes (arrows, c) and the localization of nucleolar precursor bodies (NPB) to regions of pronuclear membrane opposition are usually associated with high developmental competence

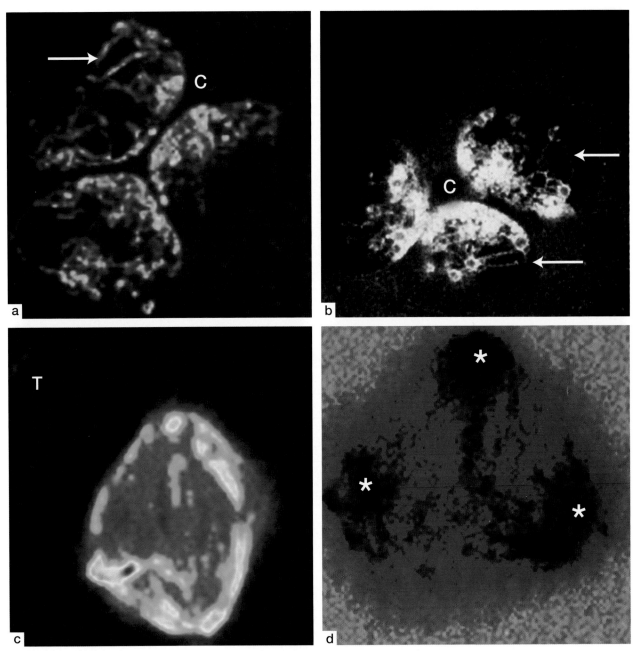

Figure 97 These scanning laser confocal images are of tripronucleate human embryos stained with a DNA-specific fluorescent probe (a, b) and anti-tubulin antibodies (d). Fluorescence imaging shows patterns of chromatin and microtubular organization that are similar to bipronuclear embryos resulting from monospermic penetration. For example, the occurrence of strands of DNA (arrows, a, b) that extend from nucleolar precursor bodies to the masses of polarized chromatin along the inner pronuclear membrane is a normal characteristic of pronuclear development in the human. In contrast to a normal bipolar mitotic spindle that develops after monospermic penetration (c), the mitotic spindle in a tripronucleate human embryo is tripolar (asterisks, d). This may account for the first cleavage division in dispermic embryos resulting in three rather than two blastomeres. The remnant of the sperm tail associated with the bipolar spindle is still evident in the normally fertilized embryo (T, c)

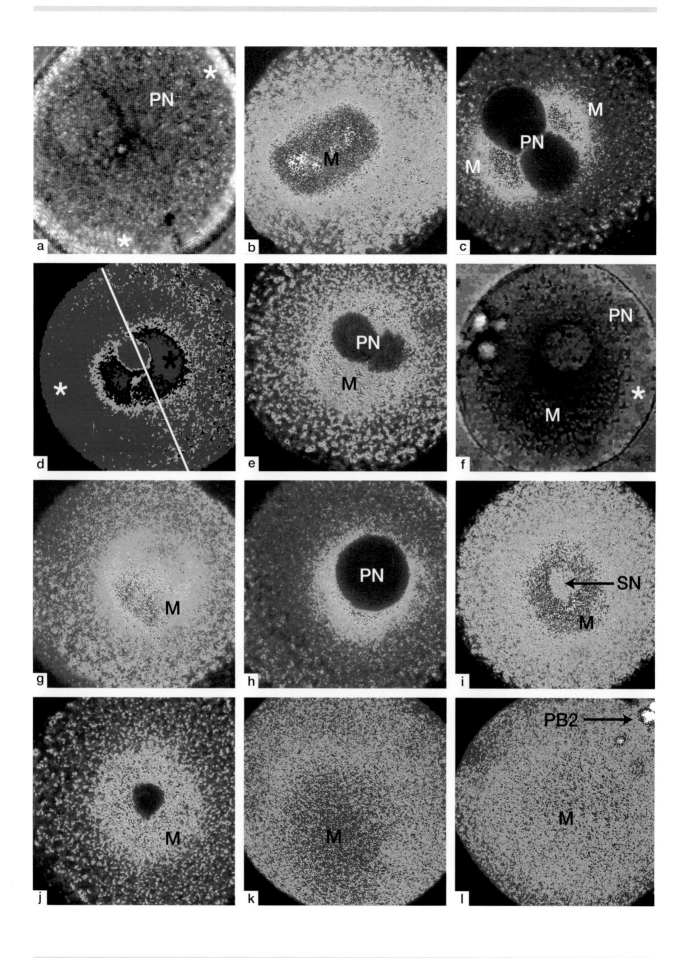

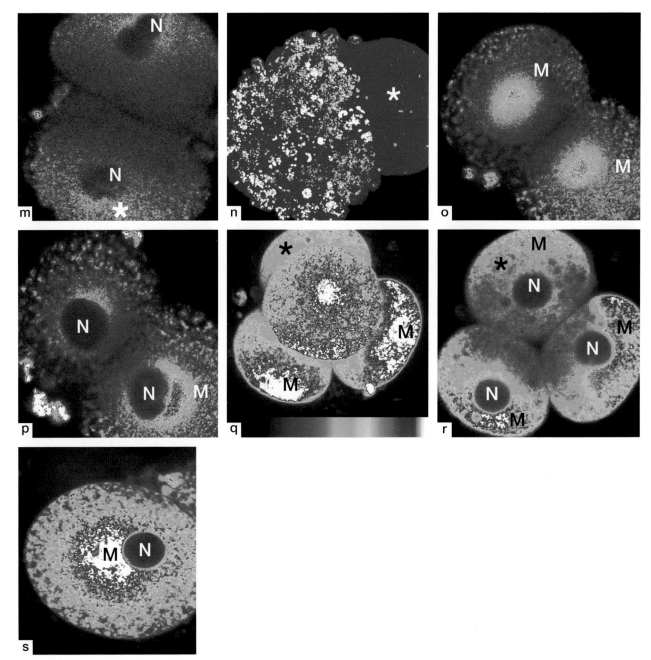

Figure 98 The pattern of peripronuclear mitochondrial aggregation is currently thought to be another dynamic aspect of cytoplasmic reorganization during the 1-cell stage of human embryogenesis that has a critical role in the normality of subsequent development. The images presented in this figure show patterns of mitochondrial distribution during the pronuclear (a–l), 2-cell (m–p) and 4-cell stages (q–s) of human preimplantation development with imaging by scanning laser confocal microscopy. Mitochondria were stained with a specific fluorescent probe and the scale bar in (q) shows the relative intensity of fluorescence from low (blue) to very high (white), which correlates with the density of mitochondria at different localizations within each cell. Normal development appears to be associated with a spherical-to-ellipsoidal aggregation of mitochondria around the pronuclei (b, c, g) which results in the inheritance of largely equivalent mitochondrial complements with each cleavage division. In contrast, an asymmetrical peripronuclear distribution (as shown in d, m, n and p) can result in disproportionate mitochondrial inheritance such that some blastomeres inherit a significantly smaller complement of these organelles. This pattern of malinheritance is seen at the 4-cell stage (q–s) by significantly different levels of mitochondrial fluorescence. The blastomere in (s) is from the 4-cell stage shown in (q) and is observed when isolated from its siblings in (r). Differences in mitochondrial inheritance in such embryos can also be seen in later stages (8–12-cell) and are associated with arrested division or cell death in blastomeres that have inherited severe numerical mitochondrial deficits. In affected cells, developmental arrest or demise has been correlated with levels of energy (ATP) production by mitochondrial oxidative phosphorylation that are insufficient to support normal developmental activities or maintain normal cellular functions and integrity

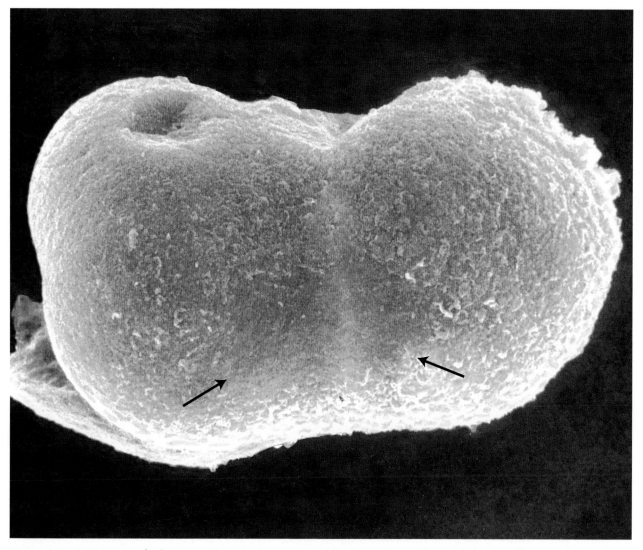

Figure 99 SEM image of a human embryo in the process of the first mitotic (cleavage) division. The arrows indicate an area between the dividing blastomeres where the surface architecture is altered by the loss of microvilli

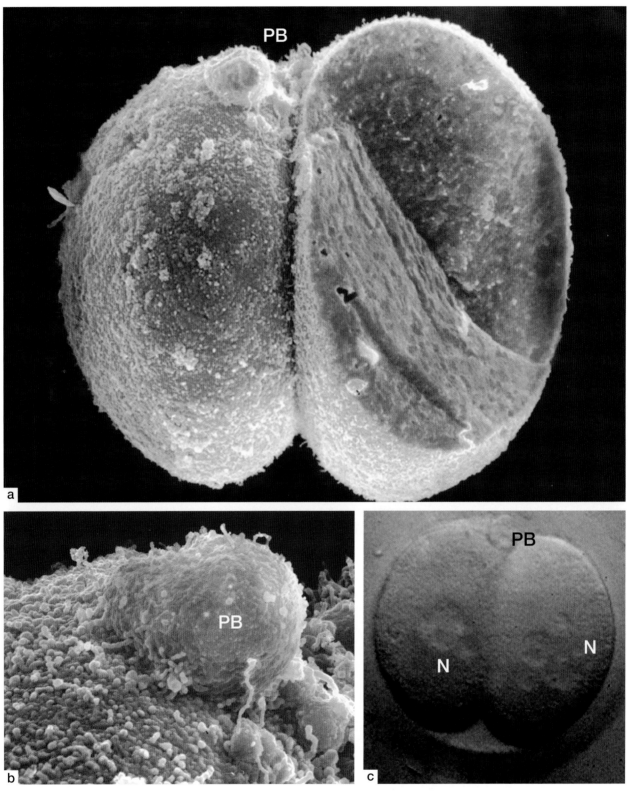

Figure 100   SEM views of a newly divided 2-cell human embryo in which one of the blastomeres was fractured to reveal the cytoplasm (a). In (b) an intact second polar body (PB) rests on the microvillous surface of one of the blastomeres. Multi- and micronucleation is a phenomenon commonly observed at the 2-cell stage in human embryos produced by IVF (c) and is developmentally lethal, because it is always associated with numerical chromosomal defects in the affected cells. N, nucleus

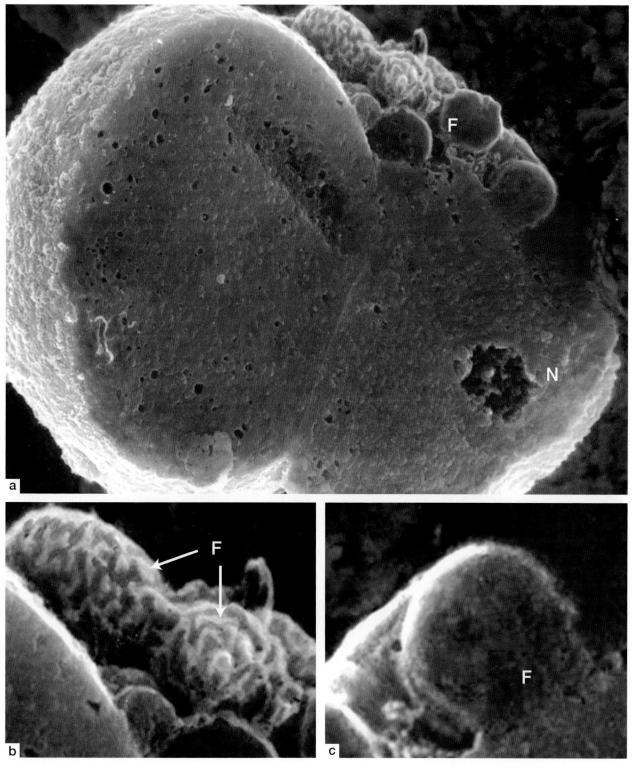

Figure 101 These SEM images of a 'fractured' 2-cell embryo show the presence of a small cluster of fragments (F) in the cleft between two blastomeres. Fragments are a common feature of cultured cleavage-stage human embryos produced by IVF and occur as a pleiomorphic population of cellular protrusions or extracellular cytoplasts, or both. Their impact on developmental competence has been associated with their number, size, distribution and composition, with toxic effects on development seen when they occur in large numbers expressed by one or both blastomeres. This is often associated with complete cellular disintegration or a significant reduction in cell volume so as to render it non-viable. In this instance, the complement of fragments is considered benign with respect to competence and for some fragments SEM imaging suggests that they are not detached but rather cytoplasmic protrusions. The occurrence of fragment-like protrusions may explain why their presence can be transitory, as time-lapse imaging demonstrates their resorption during cleavage

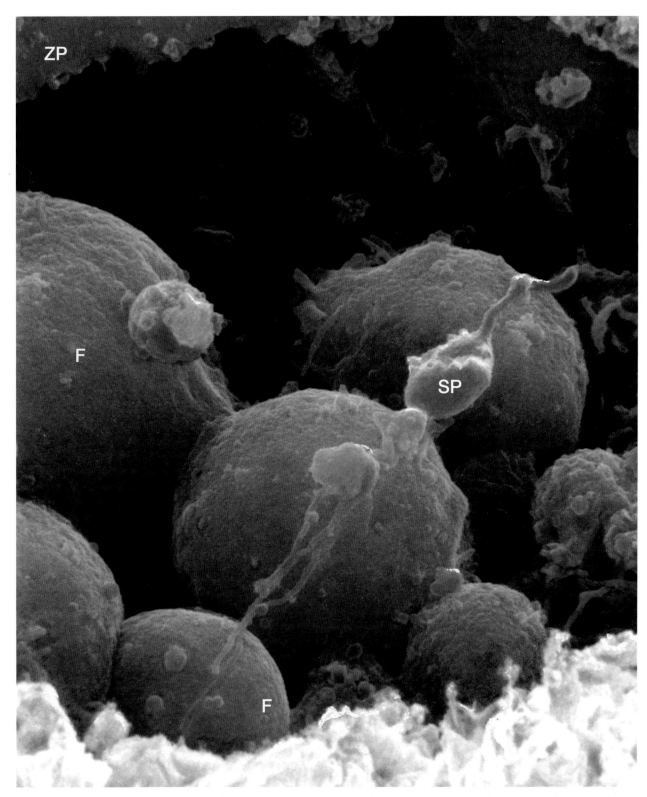

Figure 102 The pleiomorphic nature of cytoplasmic protrusions and fragments common in cleavage-stage human embryos is shown in this SEM image. In contrast to the rippled surface seen in fragments of similar density and size in Figure 101, the surface of these fragments is entirely smooth. Such differences are common when fragments are imaged by SEM and may indicate differences in the surface architecture in the region of the oolemma from which they arose, or differences in cytoplasmic composition that may manifest at the cell-surface level. Clusters of small fragments detectable by light microscopy are currently considered a normal aspect of early human embryogenesis. In this case, they may be naturally occurring cytoplasmic remnants of cell division

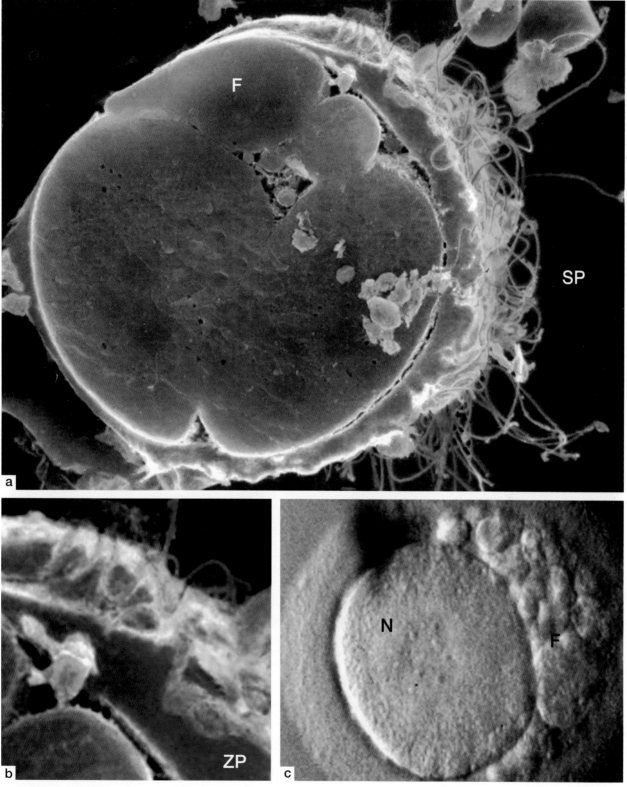

Figure 103 Occasionally, oocytes obtained from fully grown antral follicles show fragmentation patterns that are inconsistent with fertilization or, if fertilized, normal preimplantation embryogenesis (c). (a) Here, fragments of varying size are present and a sperm head on the surface of the oolemma of a small fragment is colored green and shown at higher magnification in (b). Although controversial, it has been suggested that some forms of fragmentation result from the activation of apoptotic mechanisms that prevent the fertilization or continued development of incompetent human oocytes and early embryos. Whether fragmentation at the oocyte stage is an indication of an intrinsic defect or a cellular response to abnormal intrafollicular conditions remains to be determined

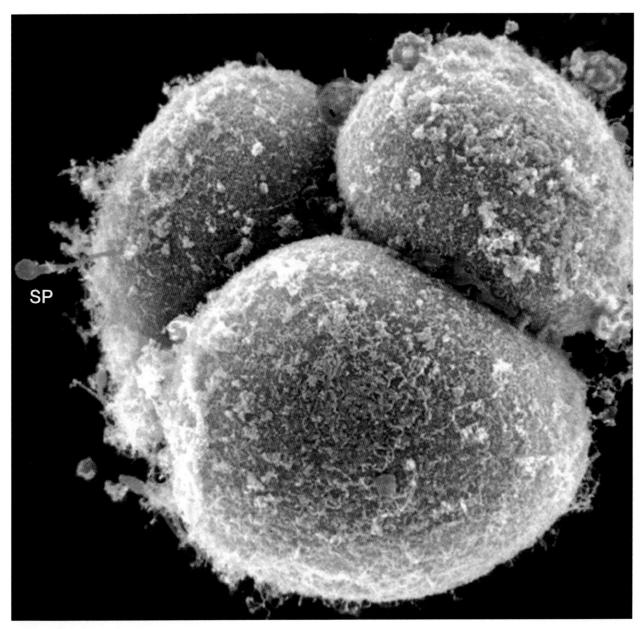

Figure 104 The timing of cleavage divisions in the early human embryo is not synchronous and, when examined after IVF, cultured embryos with odd numbers of blastomeres are observed. This figure shows a 3-cell embryo that was prepared for SEM after dissolution of the zona pellucida. The presence of blastomeres whose surface is differentially populated by microvilli and fragments is typical of early cleavage-stage human embryos. Residual spermatozoa entrapped within the zona prior to its dissolution or which had passed into the perivitelline space but did not attach to the oolemma are common in embryos obtained after conventional IVF, which involves co-culture of oocytes with thousands of spermatozoa

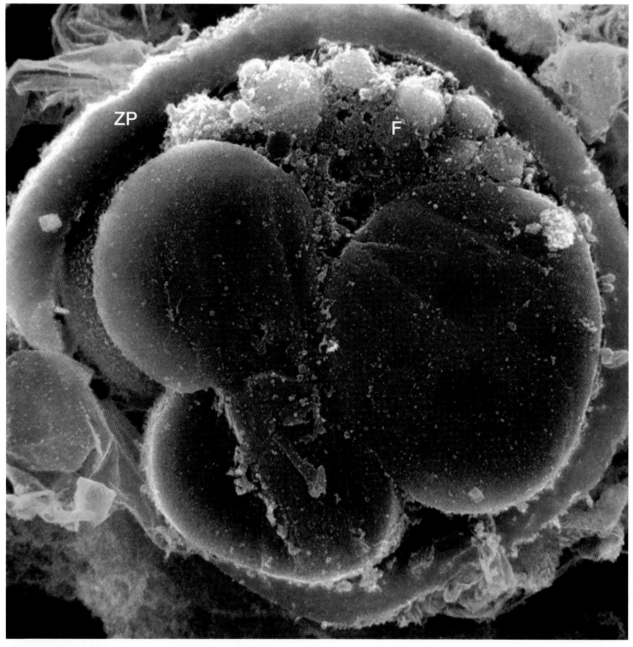

Figure 105 This image is another example of a 3-cell human embryo. In contrast to the embryo shown in Figure 104, fertilization involved intracytoplasmic sperm injection (ICSI) and SEM examination in cross section. The presence of a large cluster of fragments (F) is the most notable feature of this embryo. Embryos with this fragmentation phenotype often implant and result in normal births

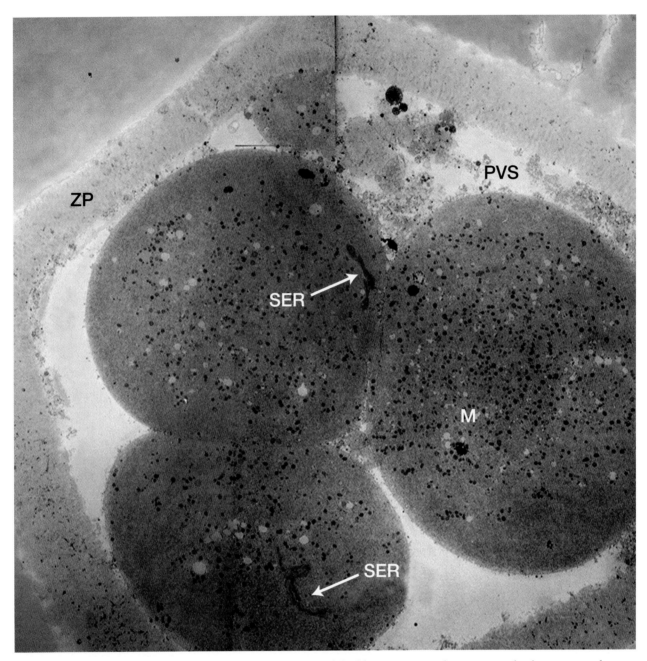

Figure 106 This TEM image shows the typical organization of the blastomere cytoplasm in an early cleavage-stage human embryo. The most notable features are the numerous spherical mitochondria (M) and long, laminar arrays of smooth-surfaced endoplasmic reticulum (SER). Typical of early human embryos is a perivitelline space (PVS) containing small cytoplasts and other membranous residues

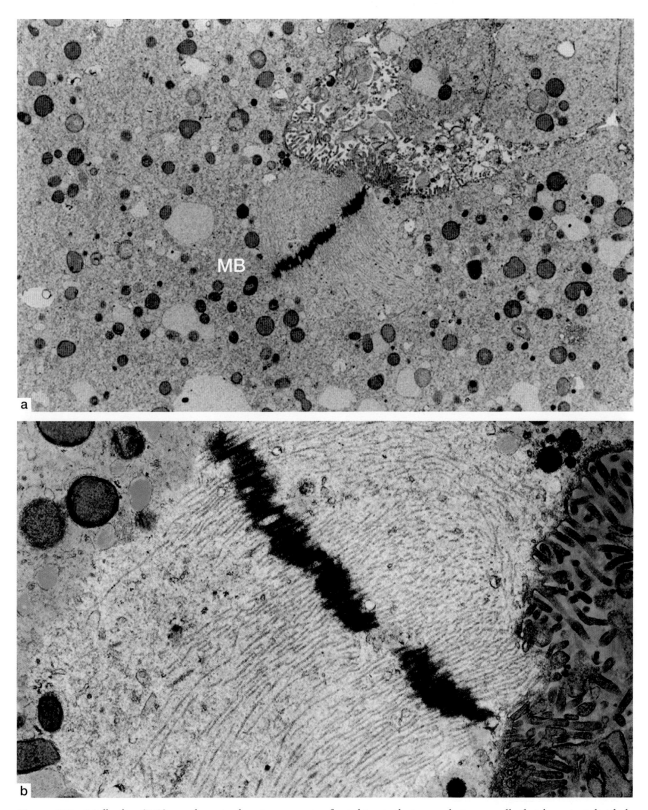

Figure 107 Midbodies (MB) are the cytoplasmic remnants of cytokinesis that occur between cells that have just divided. They are quite common in actively dividing human embryos and are defined in TEM images by the presence of arrays of microtubules left over from the mitotic spindle. Midbodies are recognized in thin sections by a characteristic dense, central band created by overlapping microtubules that is emphasized in the colorized image shown in (b). Although midbodies are cytoplasmic remnants, they contain some of the regulatory factors involved in the control of the cell cycle and may serve as an important sink for regulatory proteins whose rapid removal from daughter cells is required for normal cell-cycle timing and kinetics

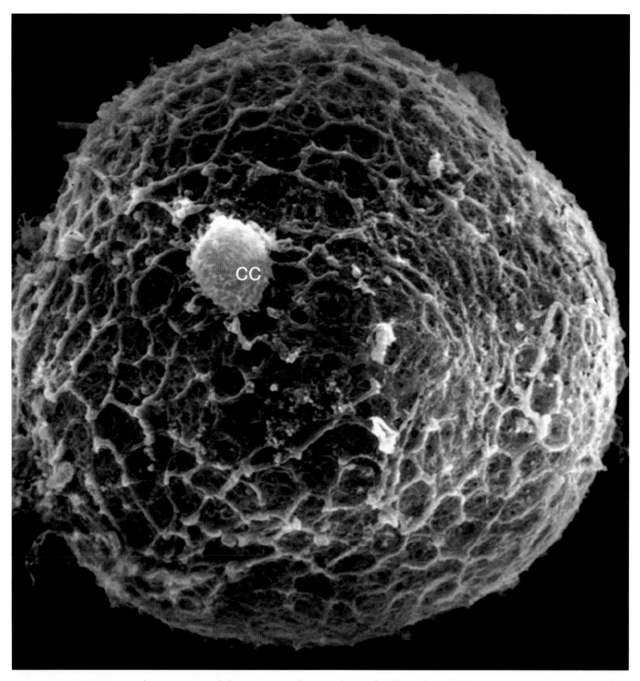

Figure 108 SEM provides a unique ability to view the topology of cells and acellular structures. Here, the surface architecture of the acellular zona pellucida in an early cleavage-stage human embryo is revealed by SEM to have a geometric arrangement that is characterized by ridge-like structures. Because this image is obtained after fixation and processing for SEM, whether this type of organization represents a state of organization that exists in the living state or is a consequence of the preparation protocol is unclear. However, the zona pellucida is known to undergo biochemical and structural changes after fertilization and differences in surface architecture seen by SEM in unfertilized oocytes, and early cleavage-stage human embryos may be manifestations of these changes, even if exaggerated by preparation for SEM. There are no accessory spermatozoa on the zona surface because fertilization involved the intracytoplasmic sperm injection of a single gamete

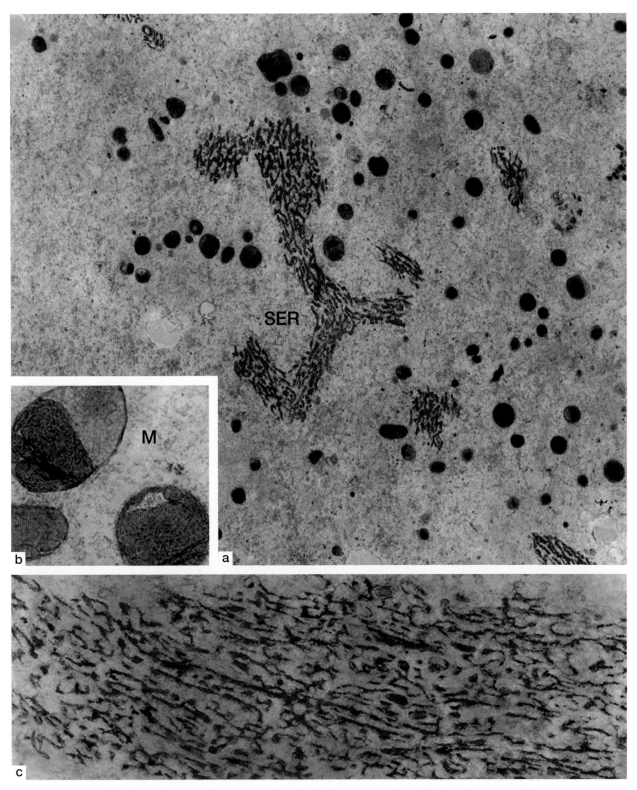

Figure 109 Mitochondria and arrays of smooth-surfaced endoplasmic reticulum (SER, a, c) are two of the most prominent features of the cytoplasm of early preimplantation-stage human embryos. Despite the fact that mitochondria appear undeveloped, owing to their spherical shape and scant cristae (b), they are metabolically active and generate ATP by oxidative phosphorylation. The SER, by virtue of its ability to sequester and release calcium, is a critical component of the early embryonic cytoplasm that is involved in calcium homeostasis and calcium-mediated regulatory processes such as the control of the cell cycle. The dense arrays of SER tubules and cisternae course through the cytoplasm. When portions of the cytoplasm are examined by serial section reconstruction, individual arrays appear to be interconnected, suggesting that SER activity may be coordinated

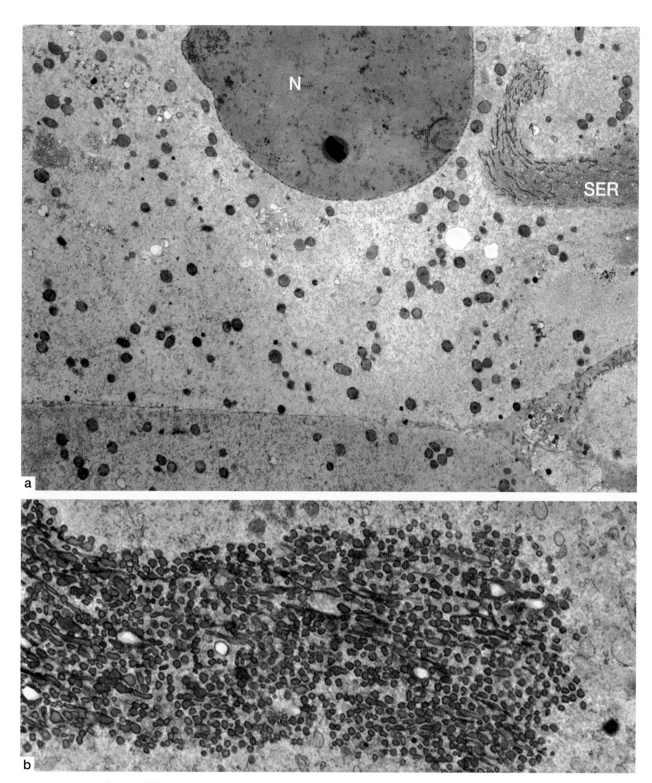

Figure 110 In this 4-cell human embryo, colorization of the SER shows a dense and enlarged array that extends from the cortical cytoplasm to the vicinity of the blastomere nucleus (N). A massive, singular array of SER tubules (b) is atypical and, if associated with defects in the regulation of intracellular free calcium, could result in developmental arrest or abnormalities if calcium-mediated regulatory and signal transduction pathways are perturbed

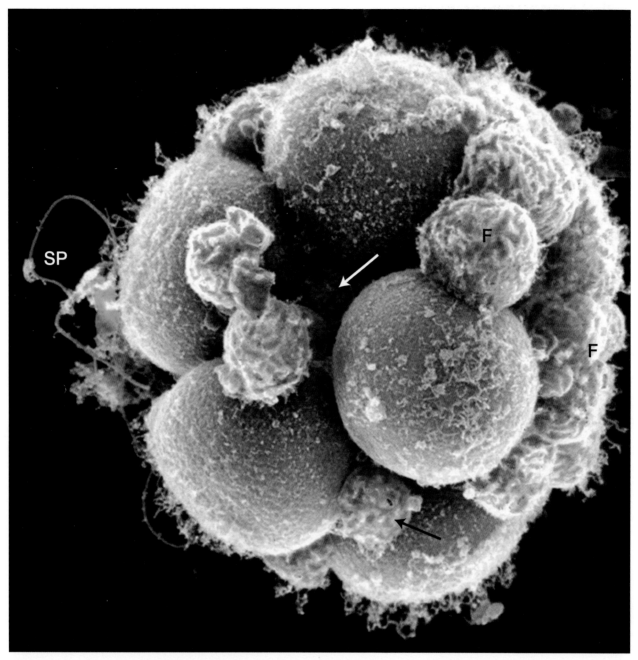

Figure 111   This image is of an 8-cell embryo in which the zona was removed prior to preparation for SEM at approximately 72 hours after conventional IVF. The 8-cell stage is especially critical for early human development because activation of the embryonic genome is thought to be largely complete, and gap-junction-mediated intercellular communication between certain blastomeres is more extensive than was seen previously. Defects in genomic activation or the establishment of channels of intercellular communication have been suggested as reasons for the early demise of human embryos. While the occurrence of extracellular fragments (F) does not necessarily indicate that the embryo would have been developmentally compromised, the internalization of fragments, such as those indicated by arrows, may present physical barriers to intercellular communication. If extensive, the occurrence of such barriers has been suggested to have negative influences on competence if they prevent the development of the widespread interactions between opposing blastomere plasma membranes that are required for the next stage in preimplantation embryogenesis: compaction

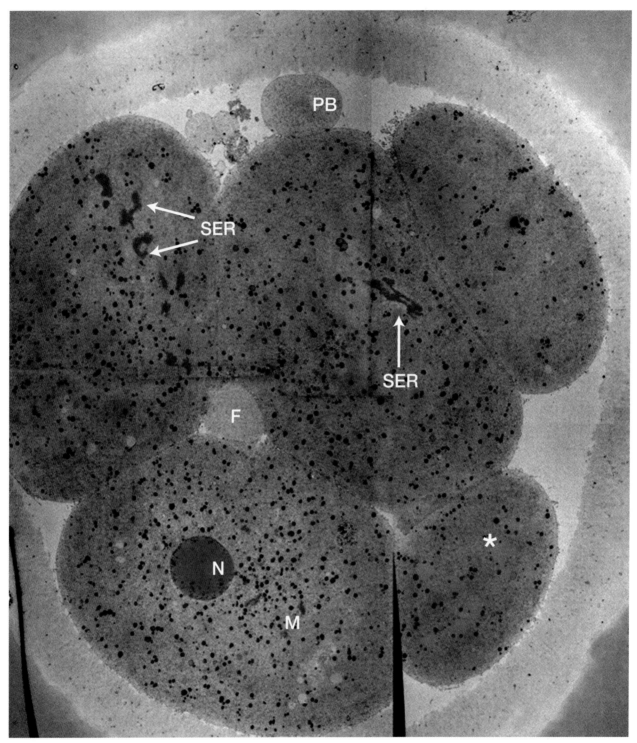

Figure 112 This TEM image indicates the typical appearance of and physical relationship between blastomeres in an 8-cell human embryo. Blastomeres can differ significantly in size and some smaller blastomeres may be large anuclear compartments (asterisk) rather than actual cells. The second polar body (PB) usually remains intact and associated with the same portion of original plasma membrane from which it emerged after fertilization. Differences in mitochondrial numbers (M) between blastomeres and putative anuclear cytoplasts that have been described by other methods are apparent in this thin section, but quantification of their numbers would require morphometric analysis. The smooth-surfaced endoplasmic reticulum (SER) persists throughout the cytoplasm in the form of densely packed arrays. This particular embryo also illustrates how internalization of extracellular fragments (F) can inhibit normal contact between blastomeres that is a hallmark of this stage of preimplantation embryogenesis

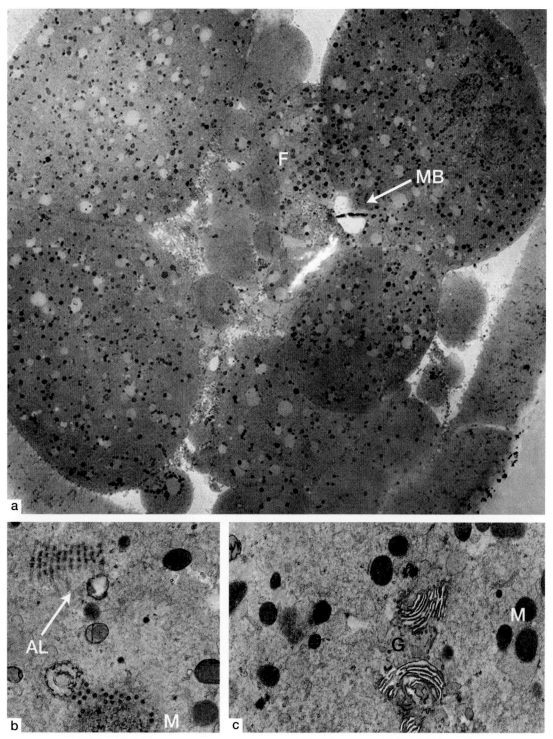

Figure 113 An example of an early cleavage-stage human embryo in which significant fragmentation has occurred during *in vitro* culture is shown in (a). TEM reveals a pleiomorphic population of extracellular fragments in which organelles such as mitochondria are largely absent or undetectable in this section. The occurrence of fragments at high density between intact blastomeres probably reflects the loss of one or more cells to fragmentation and is considered a developmentally toxic event. For the remaining blastomeres, the capacity for apparently normal cell division is suggested by the presence of a distinct midbody, although the viability of these cells cannot be determined simply by the occurrence of this structure. Cytoplasmic components normally detected by TEM in cleavage-stage human blastomeres include annulate lamellae (AL, b) and stacks of Golgi saccules (G, c), the latter of which are presumably involved in the post-translational modification of proteins destined for insertion into the plasma membrane or for secretion. Although mitochondria are metabolically active and produce ATP by oxidative phosphorylation, they remain undeveloped during the early cleavage stages as indicated by a paucity of cristae and retention of a largely spherical shape (M, b and c)

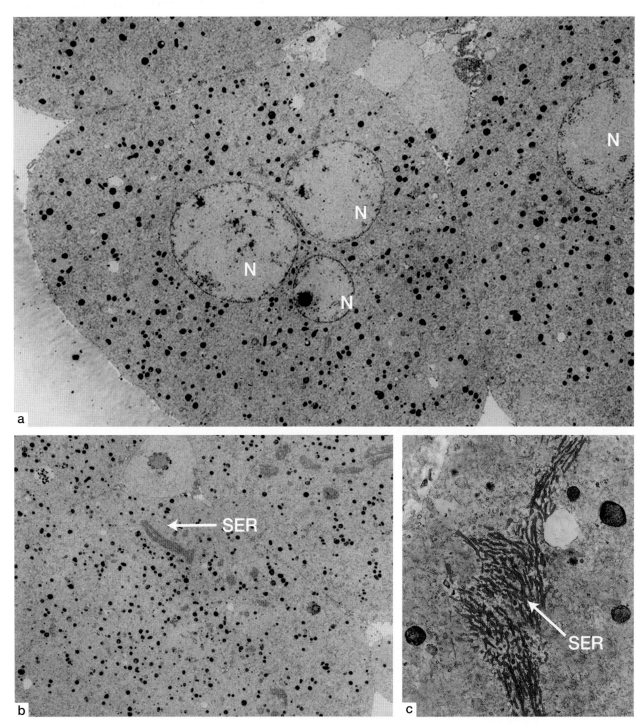

Figure 114   The presence of one or more multi- or micronucleated blastomeres is a common feature of cleavage-stage embryos produced by IVF. A blastomere from an 8-cell human embryo that appeared normal by light microscopy was found by TEM to contain three 'micronuclei' (a). The presence of a nuclear defect of this type, if restricted to one or two blastomeres, does not preclude normal embryonic development although, in clinical practice, such embryos are considered suspect. As in previous cleavage stages, arrays of SER occur throughout the cytoplasm but, unlike the oocyte, show no specific associations with mitochondria (b and c)

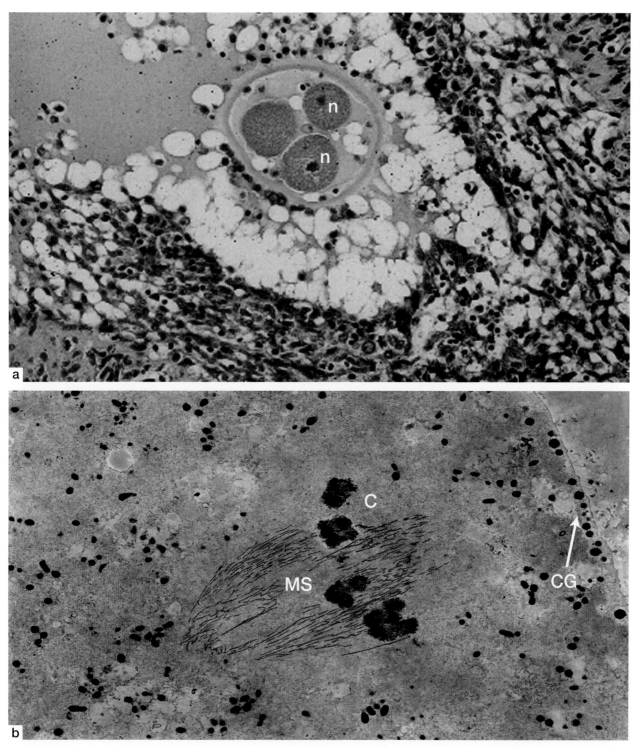

Figure 115 Occasionally, fragmented oocytes that resemble cleavage-stage embryos are observed at follicular aspiration for IVF. (a) is a light microscopic image of an antral follicle in which an apparent 4-cell embryo (three cells are shown) was observed and in which two cells were mononucleated. This phenomenon is probably the result of spontaneous (i.e. parthenogenetic) activation and it is likely that ovarian teratomas arise from oocytes such as this. (b) shows a putative mitotic spindle (MS) in a 2-cell parthenogenetic embryo that was recovered at aspiration from a fully grown antral follicle. A parthenogenetic origin is further indicated by the retention of cortical granules (CG). C, chromosome

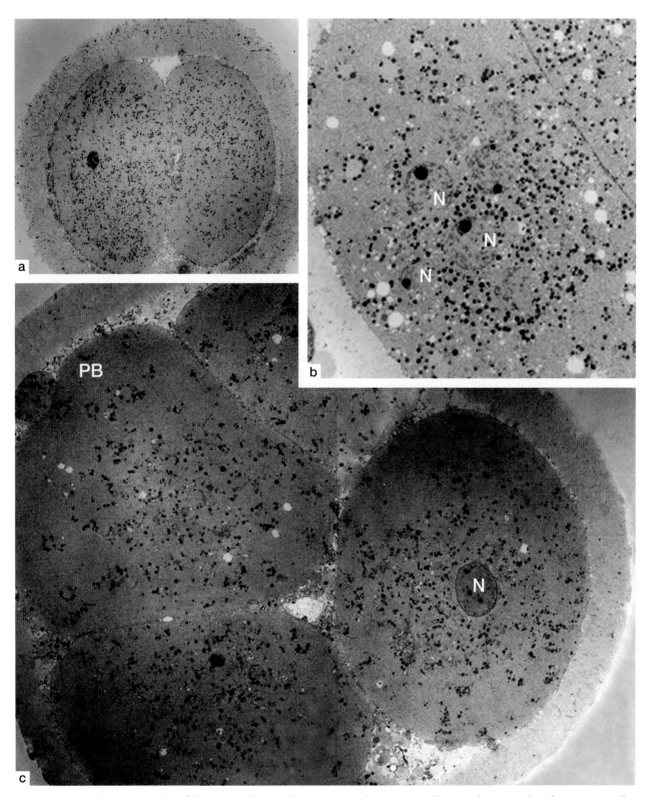

Figure 116 Other examples of human embryos that arose parthenogenetically are show in this figure. Typically, spontaneous parthenogenesis in the human results in cleavage-stage embryos that contain mononucleated (c) and micronucleated blastomeres (b). By TEM, blastomeres in 2-cell embryos (a) through the cleavage stages (6-cell, c) are very similar to their counterparts in normally fertilized embryos. Indeed, under certain circumstances, some human embryos derived by spontaneous or experimentally induced parthenogenesis can develop to the hatched blastocyst stage. N, nucleus; PB, polar body

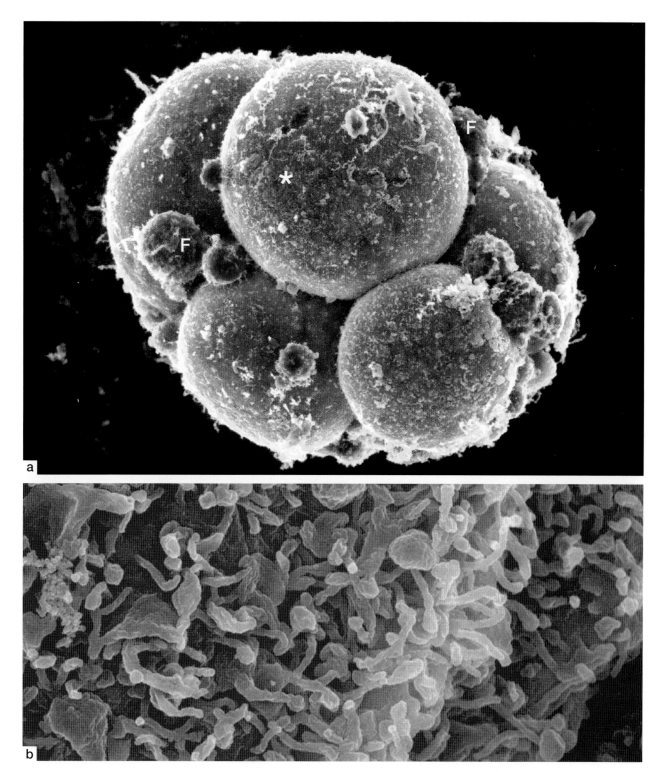

Figure 117 An 8-cell human parthenogenetic embryo derived from a metaphase II-stage oocyte that underwent spontaneous activation *in vitro* is shown in this colorized SEM image. By SEM, cell-surface architecture and the presence of a few extracellular fragments (F) are the same features encountered in normal 8-cell embryos. For example, a dense population of microvilli is a characteristic feature of a normally fertilized 8-cell human embryo. The microvillous region of a blastomere surface shown in (b) (taken from the region indicated by an asterisk in a) is indistinguishable from a similar region that would be observed in a normal embryo. At this stage of development and at this level of resolution, the presence of a paternal (sperm) genome does not appear to be required for or associated with the expression of a cell-surface organization that is stage-specific

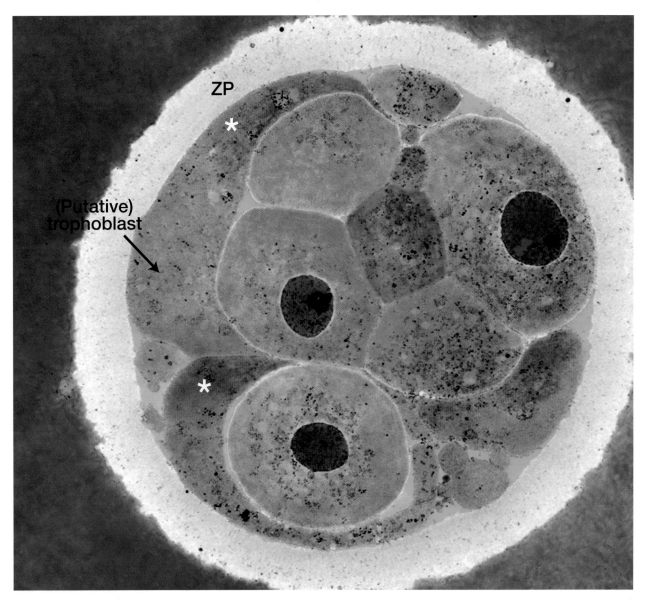

Figure 118 After the 14–16-cell stage of human development, embryos undergo a morphodynamic process termed compaction, whereby the close opposition of blastomere cell membranes obscures the borders between cells. Compaction is essential for normal embryogenesis as it permits the initial establishment of the two basic cell lineages of the preimplantation-stage embryo: the trophectoderm and the inner cell mass. The external cells normally give rise to the trophectoderm (also termed the trophoblast) that ultimately develops into the extraembryonic membranes and placenta. Internal cells form the inner cell mass from which the embryo proper will develop. This colorized TEM image of an early stage of compaction shows the close apposition of opposing cell membranes and the occurrence of cells that are either relatively spherical or elongated. The elongated cells colored blue are likely to form the trophectoderm and here are noted as putative trophoblast. Some of the blastomeres colored orange will form the inner cell mass, but specific designations as to developmental fate cannot be made for individual cells in this embryo. The morphodynamic nature of the compaction process is indicted by the two 'trophoblast' cells denoted by an asterisk. These cells appear to be in the process of enclosing the internal cells and for the cell in the lower portion of the figure, serial section reconstructions demonstrate that the interior cell (orange colored) is partially engulfed by the outer cell. This morphodynamic phenomenon resembling an engulfment process is transient because, as development through the morula stage progresses, the outer cells become elongated whereas the shape of the inner cells that develop into the inner cell mass remain largely spherical, as shown in Figure 119

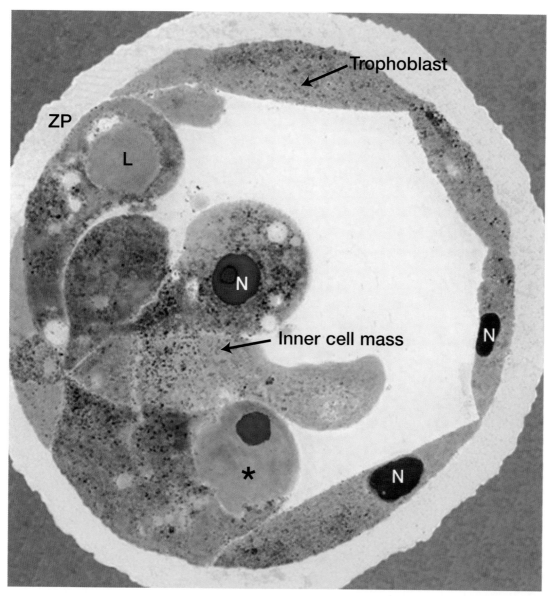

Figure 119 The accumulation of fluid within the interior of the compacted embryo is a second fundamental event that occurs during the morula stage, and one that is essential for normal embryogenesis and progression to the blastocyst stage. The development of tight junctions and desmosomes between the outer (trophoblast) cells forms an effective seal that permits fluid accumulation within the embryo. The developing trophoblast cells are highly specialized with multiple functions, one of which is to serve as a transporting epithelium. In this capacity, the apical surface of the forming trophoblast takes up fluid from the perivitelline space by endocytosis and, by means of unidirectional vesicular traffic, deposits fluid internally by exocytosis from the basal surface. The accumulation of fluid within the internal aspect of the embryo defines a process termed cavitation, whereby a progressively enlarging, fluid-filled cavity develops.

In this colorized TEM image of an early cavitation-stage human embryo, the accumulated fluid is shown in blue. The progressive expansion of the cavity flattens the outer trophoblast cells. Fluid does not escape, owing to tight junctions between trophoblast cells, while internally they develop desmosomes whose associated arrays of microfilaments extend from one end of the cell to the other. This filamentous network provides an internal skeleton that is thought to enable the cells to withstand the physical forces generated by fluid accumulation that results in their becoming highly flattened. The typical elongated/flattened shape of trophoblast cells is already evident in this early cavitating embryo. In contrast, cells of the developing inner cell mass (ICM) remain relatively round during this early expansion phase.

Although this appeared by light microscopy to be a normally developing late morula-stage embryo, TEM analysis shows apparent abnormalities in the structure and organization of the ICM, but not the trophoblast, that would seem to be inconsistent with normal embryogenesis. For example, while the trophoblast cells appear normal in composition and organization, some of the ICM cells show degenerative characteristics indicated by large lipid bodies (L), vesicles and (anuclear) cytoplasts (asterisk). If implanted, it is likely that embryos of this type (so-called blighted ova) result in anembryonic pregnancies in which placental structures develop in the absence of a fetus

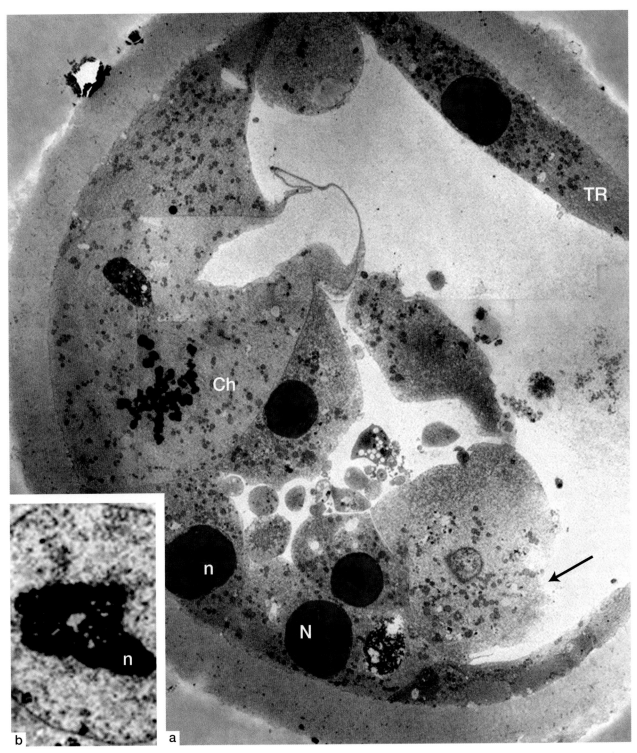

Figure 120 With continued fluid accumulation, the embryo transforms from a cavitating morula to an expanding blastocyst. The enlarging fluid-filled cavity is termed the blastocyst cavity or blastocoel. (a) This TEM image of an expanding human blastocyst is another example of abnormal development during the latter stages of human preimplantation embryogenesis. The ICM appears unorganized and contains fragmented and lysed (arrow) cells. However, indications of cell viability are suggested for some cells visible in this thin section by the presence of fully differentiated nucleoli (a, b) that presumably are actively engaged in the transcription of transfer and ribosomal RNA. It is unclear whether the putative trophoblast (TR) cell containing a mass of chromosomes (Ch) within the cytoplasm is either normal or viable. N, nucleus

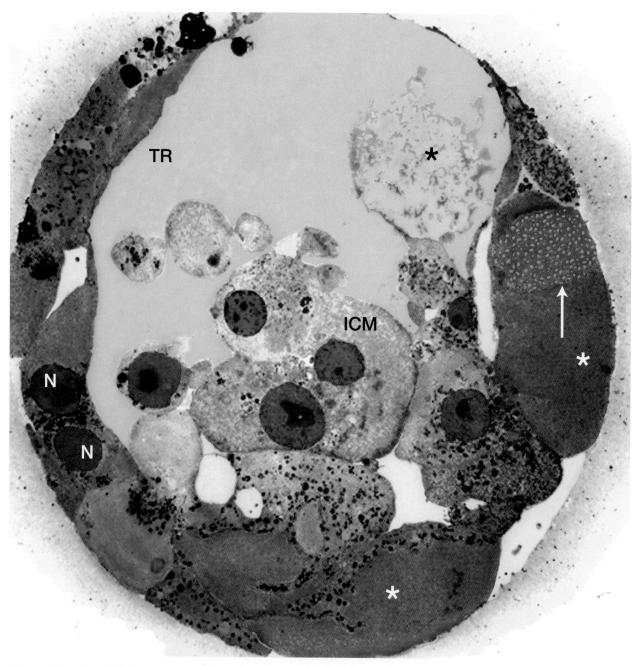

Figure 121 This TEM image shows the fine structural characteristics of an early blastocyst-stage human embryo that arrested expansion and development after approximately 5 days of culture. In this instance, not only is the ICM disorganized, a common feature of developmentally compromised human blastocysts, but, unlike other examples of apparently non-viable blastocysts shown previously, the trophoblast (TR) is composed of cells with few organelles, with no detectable nuclei (indicated by white asterisks), or which are multinucleated (cell at far left, for example). The remnants of a lysed inner cell mass cell are indicated by a black asterisk. One of the common features of preimplantation human embryogenesis *in vitro* is that blastocyst-like embryos can form with fewer than 20 cells, in contrast to the hundred or more normally present in a 5- or 6-day-old embryo. This embryo appears to be an example of such a phenomenon and is equally remarkable for developing and maintaining a blastocoel with trophoblast cells that are so aberrant. Chromosomal abnormalities associated with nuclear defects, such as the binucleated trophoblast cell shown here, is another common feature of human blastocysts. However, their occurrence in otherwise normally developing embryos is not currently thought to preclude normal births

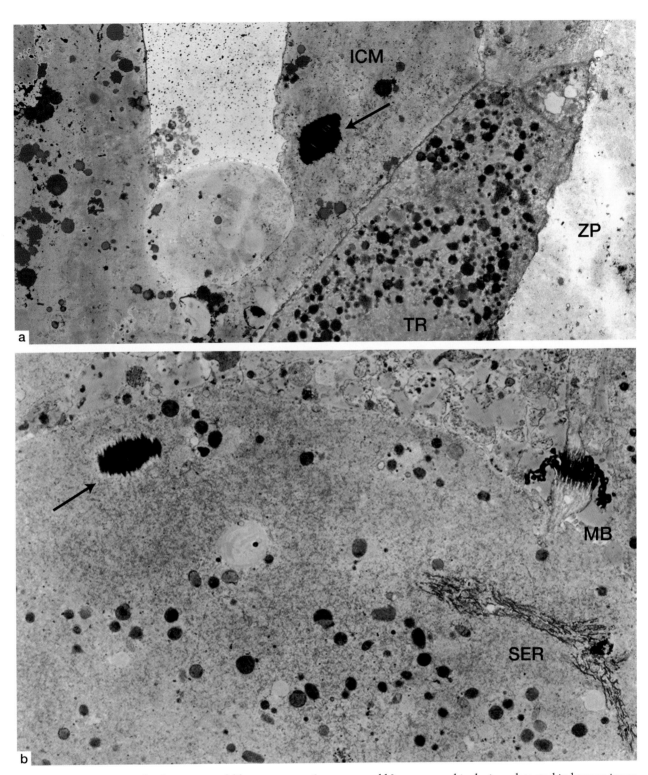

Figure 122 Structures that have a crystal-like appearance (arrows, a and b) are unusual inclusions detected in human inner cell mass cells at the blastocyst stage (a) and in blastomeres during cleavage (b). Although their composition is unknown, they are often detected in cells containing a midbody (MB, b) and could represent certain proteins whose presence at high concentration in a particular region of the cytoplasm leads to self-assembly into paracrystalline structures

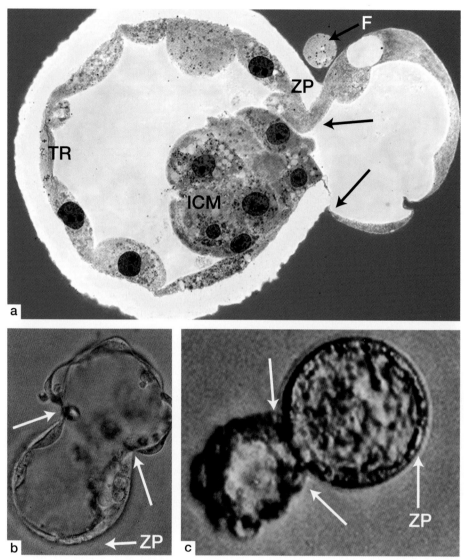

Figure 123 Approximately 6 to 6.5 days after fertilization, the blastocyst-stage embryo emerges from the zona pellucida by a process commonly termed 'hatching'. Hatching involves the creation of a rent in the zona pellucida by enzymatic digestion and physical disruption mediated by specialized filapodia elaborated by certain trophoblast cells. Emergence of the embryo through the rent involves mechanical forces generated by the expanding blastocyst. It is thought that some cases of monozygotic and conjoined twins result from a complete or partial splitting of the embryo, respectively, if the hole in the zona is unusually small, which may create atypical shearing forces during the hatching process. Light microscopic views of living normal human blastocysts photographed in the process of emerging from within the zona pellucida (ZP) are shown in (b and c). The region of dissolved zona pellucida through which the embryos are emerging is indicated by arrows. Emergence is a relatively rapid process and is a perquisite for implantation. Failure to hatch has been considered one reason for the inability of seemingly normal blastocysts to implant after uterine transfer. This notion has led to the development of several manipulative techniques, commonly known as 'assisted hatching', which create an artificial rent in the zona in order to ensure that an exit for the embryos exists. Although controversial, outcome data suggest that this may be beneficial in the following instances: (1) certain cases of infertility, such as in women of advanced reproductive age, or where multiple IVF attempts with normal-appearing embryos have failed; or (2) with thawed embryos where cryopreservation may have artifactually 'hardened' the zona pellucida, making it resistant to the normal physical and enzymatic mechanisms the embryo employs to emerge.

The colorized TEM image in (a) shows a normal human blastocyst fixed at the moment that the portion of the embryo containing the inner cell mass (ICM) is just about to emerge. In contrast to previous images of blastocysts, note the compact and intact nature of the ICM, the elongated organization of the trophoblast (TR) and the apparent absence of cytoplasmic defects or indications of cellular degeneration in both cell types. The presence of small extracellular cytoplasmic fragments (F) is a common occurrence in hatching human blastocysts and probably represents residual structures that were elaborated during cleavage. The region of the zona pellucida through which the embryo is emerging is delineated between the two arrows

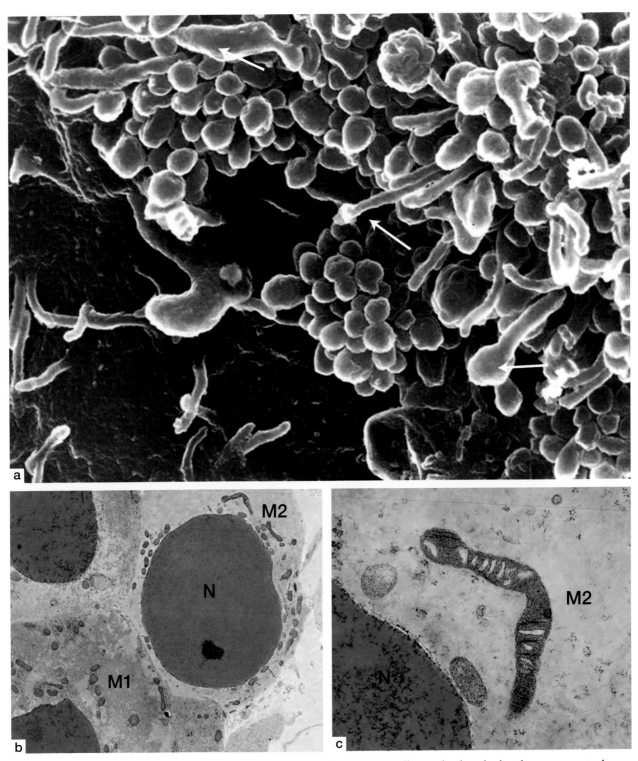

Figure 124 The surface of the trophoblast in the region of a blastocyst initially involved in the hatching process is shown in this SEM image (a). The elongated filopodia indicated by arrows are of particular interest as they may have been involved in assisting the local dissolution of the zona pellucida. Focal regions containing elongated filopodia of this type are involved in hatching in other mammals, and the term 'zona breaker' has recently been used to describe their function in the human. Changes in mitochondrial structure and organization are one of the characteristic subcellular features evident in blastocyst-stage human embryos. (b and c) show the occurrence of two mitochondrial phenotypes, labeled M1 and M2, in an expanded blastocyst. Although most still retain the spherical profile typical of previous stages (M1), others show the 'orthodox' form in which mitochondria are elongated and contain numerous cristae completely traversing the inner matrix (M2). Traditionally, orthodox forms are associated with higher levels of activity, including the generation of ATP by oxidative phosphorylation

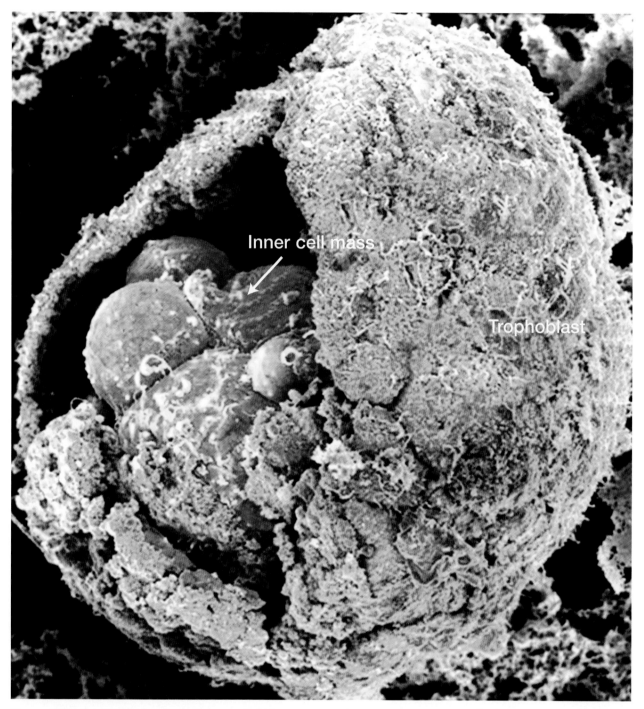

Figure 125 For this SEM analysis, the expanded blastocyst-stage human embryo was partially fractured after processing to reveal the inner cell mass (ICM). As known from light and TEM imaging, the ICM cells in a normal blastocyst exist as an intact and well-defined cluster of large, round cells. It is from the ICM that the fetus develops and it is therefore not surprising that the same cells are used to derive totipotential stem cells

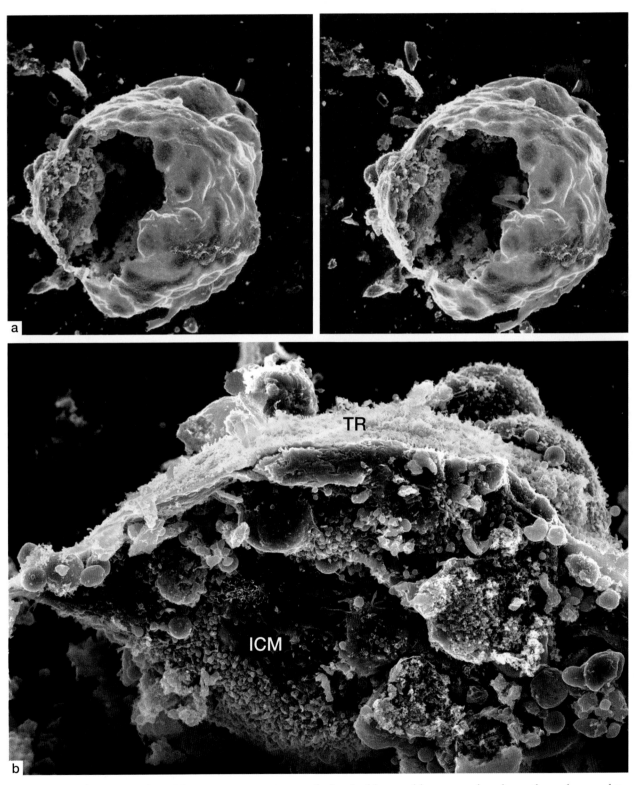

Figure 126 The two panels in (a) are a stereo-pair image of a hatched human blastomere that shows the embryo and its ICM in a three-dimensional aspect when using the crossed eyes method. (b) shows the portion of the same embryo containing the ICM and overlying trophoblast, which is colored blue. The green-colored protrusions on the trophoblast may be cells in mitosis

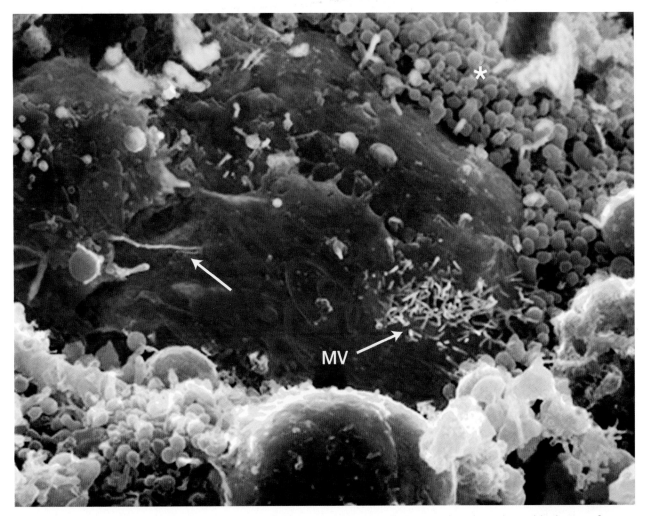

Figure 127 The power of SEM in the analysis of human embryos is well illustrated in this colorized high-magnification image of the ICM in the embryo shown in Figure 126. Regional differences in surface architecture within the ICM range from smooth-surfaced cells to those adorned with clumps of microvilli (MV) or a dense population of small, bleb-like bodies (asterisk). The presence of blebs is currently thought to be indicative of secretory activity, although this notion will need biochemical confirmation. Elongated cellular protrusions (arrow) extending between ICM cells are considered a normal aspect of a competent ICM and their detection by high-resolution light microscopy is one of the morphological characteristics of expanded blastocysts used to assess embryos for transfer after IVF. The occurrence of these projections may reflect a migratory ability for some cells within the ICM. The diversity of surface morphologies in the ICM is one of the more unexpected findings to come from SEM analysis of human blastocysts

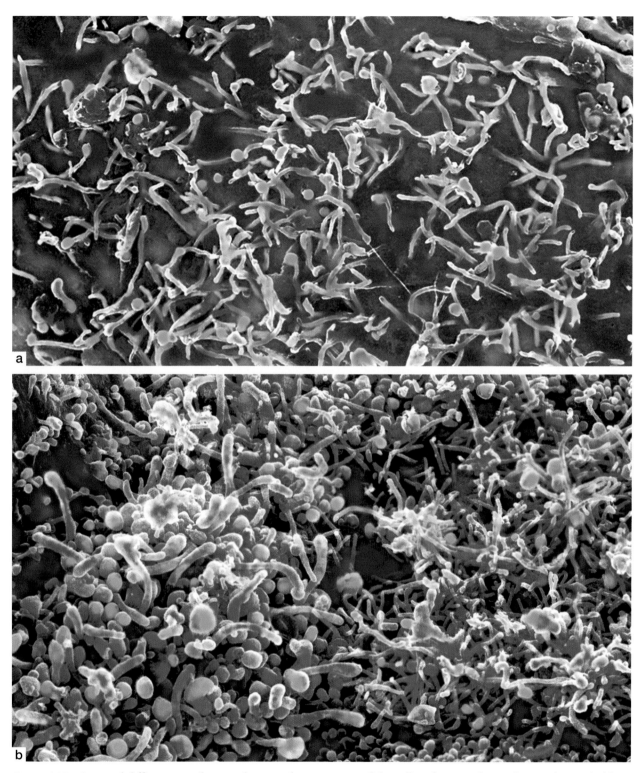

Figure 128 Regional differences in the complexity and organization of the cell surface are also evident in the trophoblast. While some trophoblast cells are adorned by microvilli (a), other regions contain a dense array of secretory-type protrusions and blebs intermingled with microvilli (b). Regional differences in surface architecture within the trophoblast may reflect corresponding differences in cell function or activity. For example, trophoblast cells export a diverse array of growth factors, cytokines and adhesion-mediating molecules that are currently believed to arise from those cells with a bleb-like component. Although speculative at present, it is an intriguing possibility that regional differences do reflect functional differences. For example, perhaps the secretory/microvillous domains are involved in the attachment of the embryo to the endometrial epithelium

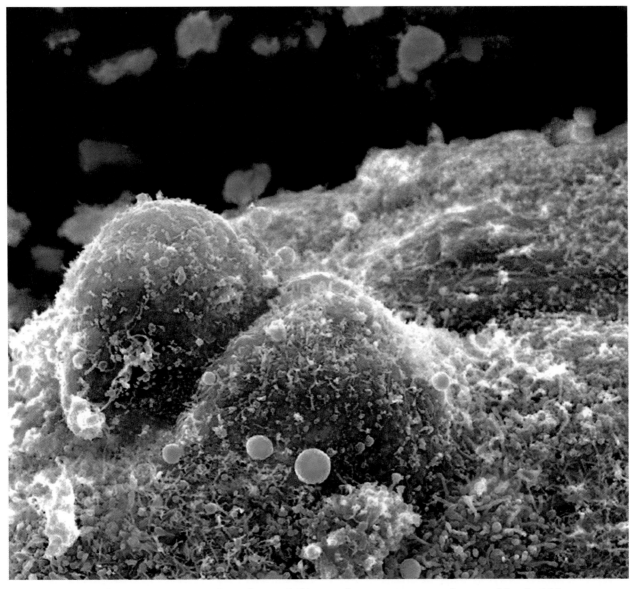

Figure 129 Paired protrusions arising from the trophoblast surface are a common feature of hatched blastocyst-stage human embryos. Although their origin is unknown, it is currently believed that they represent a portion of cells undergoing division and their presence is indicative of a normal trophoblast

Index